'People living with Parkinson's
can make lifestyle changes to live
physical activity, following a ba
wellbeing can all have a positive
based book provides an excell   ... to help people with
Parkinson's take up and maintain healthy habits.'

Claire Bale, *Associate Director of Research, Parkinson's UK*

LIVING WELL WITH PARKINSON'S

This accessible guide provides evidence-based approaches to support those with Parkinson's. It offers a roadmap to not only managing the symptoms but also thriving with the condition, allowing individuals and their care partners to develop a comprehensive approach to living well with Parkinson's, emphasising proactive engagement with healthcare professionals, emotional resilience, and achievable goals.

The book begins by providing a clear understanding of Parkinson's, including its diagnosis, causes, progression, and various symptoms. It then delves into the impact of the disease on a person's health and well-being, focusing on non-motor symptoms, mental health, and daily life adjustments. This guide explores practical strategies for nurturing relationships with family and friends, providing insights into maintaining emotional connections and communication during the journey with Parkinson's. Furthermore, the book delves into self-care aspects, addressing how individuals can take control of their health through sleep improvement, nutrition, physical activity, and relaxation techniques. Readers will discover a holistic approach to well-being, emphasising the significance of these factors in managing Parkinson's effectively.

The book serves as a valuable companion for those navigating the complex terrain of Parkinson's, offering hope, knowledge, and practical guidance on the journey to living a rich, meaningful, and fulfilling life.

Angeliki Bogosian is a health psychologist and academic working at City, St George's University of London, UK. Her research is at the forefront of practice. She has a nationally established profile in leading interdisciplinary studies identifying effective and cost-effective ways to give people with long-term conditions the tools to manage physical and psychological challenges. She specialises in acceptance and commitment therapies and mindfulness training and works mainly with people with neurological conditions.

BPS ASK THE EXPERTS IN PSYCHOLOGY SERIES

British Psychological Society

Routledge, in partnership with the British Psychological Society (BPS), is pleased to present BPS Ask the Experts, a new popular science series that addresses key issues and answers the burning questions. Drawing on the expertise of established psychologists, every book in the series provides authoritative and straightforward guidance on pressing topics that matter to real people in their everyday lives.

All books in the BPS Ask the Experts series are written for the reader with no prior knowledge or experience. For answers to everything you ever wanted to know about issues important to you, ask the expert!

For more information about this series, please visit: BPS Ask The Experts in Psychology Series – Book Series – Routledge & CRC Press

LIVING WELL WITH PARKINSON'S

A Guide to a Fulfilling Life

ANGELIKI BOGOSIAN

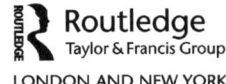

Routledge
Taylor & Francis Group

LONDON AND NEW YORK

Designed cover image: Getty Images

First published 2026
by Routledge
4 Park Square, Milton Park, Abingdon, Oxon OX14 4RN

and by Routledge
605 Third Avenue, New York, NY 10158

Routledge is an imprint of the Taylor & Francis Group, an informa business

British Library Cataloguing-in-Publication Data
A catalogue record for this book is available from the British Library

ISBN: 978-1-032-77684-2 (hbk)
ISBN: 978-1-032-77682-8 (pbk)
ISBN: 978-1-003-48433-2 (ebk)

DOI: 10.4324/9781003484332

Typeset in Bembo
by Apex CoVantage, LLC

Access the Support Material: www.routledge.com/9781032776828

CONTENTS

WHO AM I AND WHY AM I GIVING YOU THIS ADVICE?

Can you live a healthy, happy life after a diagnosis of Parkinson's? Can you go from feeling anxious about the future to enjoying your present? From having Parkinson's symptoms taking up all your mental and physical energy to creating a life where you focus on the things you want and are important to you? This book will discuss psychological science, which shows how to achieve these changes. You may not have control over Parkinson's symptoms, thoughts, or feelings, but the techniques I will discuss here will help you control their impact on your life.

Living with Parkinson's provides a complex and multifaceted journey: a journey that demands flexibility, resilience, and a holistic approach to well-being. As the journey with Parkinson's unfolds, you may encounter not only physical symptoms but also emotional, social, and practical hurdles that require navigation and understanding.

A common advice doctors give to people diagnosed with a long-term condition, that is, a condition that cannot be cured but symptoms can be managed, is to lead a healthy lifestyle, becoming more conscious about what sustains good physical and mental health and maintaining it. As someone with Parkinson's once told me, 'With Parkinson's, I have to be double healthy'. This will help the body

DOI: 10.4324/9781003484332-1

manage the Parkinson's symptoms and prevent further long-term conditions, which are sure to complicate your day-to-day life. Enhancing and maintaining your general health will involve healthy eating, physical activity, managing stress, and adhering to medication plans. These behaviours will not only help you keep healthy but also positively affect your mental health, and good mental health will support you in managing motor and non-motor symptoms and maintaining overall good physical health.

In this book, I will draw on my expertise as a health psychologist to discuss behaviour-change techniques that can help you maintain good health habits and let go of habits that don't serve your health goals. Health psychology is a discipline that focuses on supporting people in changing their health-related behaviours and managing common long-term condition symptoms, such as pain, sleep difficulties, and fatigue.

My research focuses on well-being and neurological conditions. I have conducted numerous research projects, looking at factors that influence psychological well-being and developing and testing well-being programmes for people with multiple sclerosis and Parkinson's and their families. I have published more than 30 articles in medical and psychological scientific journals. I have also written a book on how to live well with a long-term condition, where I discuss general principles on managing common physical symptoms and how to lead a full and meaningful life.

Here, I will narrow down the focus and talk about Parkinson's and discuss how you can lead a full and meaningful life despite the challenges Parkinson's brings. I will also go a step further and say that Parkinson's could be one of those transformative experiences. Even though it comes with many challenges that cannot be ignored or underestimated, it might also enable you to re-assess priorities, reflect on what is important to you, and look at how your life aligns with your priorities. Here, I will discuss what we know about Parkinson's and Parkinson's symptoms. Then, I will discuss ways to increase emotional resilience and align your goals with what you do everyday. If I were to observe you all day, would I be able to guess your values by your actions?

I will delve into various aspects of life affected by Parkinson's, from managing emotions, fostering meaningful relationships, and navigating daily activities. I will also discuss managing common symptoms like pain, fatigue, and mild cognitive difficulties. Finally, I will cover some habits that support your physical health (like healthy eating and physical activity) and ways to incorporate those in your life. Whether you're newly diagnosed or diagnosed a long time ago or someone walking alongside someone on this journey, 'Living Well with Parkinson's' offers guidance, support, and hope for a life lived to its fullest potential.

1

WHAT IS PARKINSON'S?

Patrick was in shock when he got the Parkinson's diagnosis; he was told he had Parkinson's, and that was it. He expected someone from the hospital or general practitioner (GP) surgery to get in touch to explain further and give him some guidance, but nobody did. Having Parkinson's was hard, but he was trying to focus on the present, on the day ahead and not worry too much about the future. He had to take a lot of medication now at various times of the day, and he wasn't feeling comfortable with this. He had always resisted taking medication about anything. He had read through all the information about each tablet to spot any side effects and weigh the pros and cons. He was setting alarms to make sure he took his tablets on time. Parkinson's meant he could not do things that he once took for granted, like negotiating stairs, doing the weekly food shop or cooking. Despite this, he still feels like him. He's still a father, a husband, and a volunteer for his local park. He sometimes felt embarrassed when he was out and about. He felt people were watching and judging him, mistaking him for being drunk. He had discussed this with his wife and tried not to let this get in the way of him living his life. They've been going out for short walks into the town every day, and it has become a way to connect with his wife and keep his body moving. To manage the off periods and the

DOI: 10.4324/9781003484332-2

fatigue and also to make sure he sees his son and his grandkids, he was now asking them to visit him at home, so if he felt he needed some rest, he could go upstairs to his bedroom, and his family will be understanding.

What you thought you knew about Parkinson's when you were first diagnosed is not what you know now. Parkinson's is a common neurological condition, and yet it is misunderstood by many. We associate Parkinson's with tremors, but there is an array of symptoms that can be more or less distressing for individuals. But let's start from the beginning.

Two hundred years ago, at age 62, James Parkinson (1755–1824) wrote a 66-page treatise titled 'An Essay on the Shaking Palsy' (Parkinson, 1817), in which he described six clinical vignettes. We mark his birthday every 11 April with World Parkinson's Day, a day to shine a spotlight on Parkinson's. Lees et al. (2017) in *Brain Journal* describes the vignettes as 'easy to read and as refreshing as wine'. This essay, with the six vignettes, was the first document that described the condition, even though we did not have the technology to understand how it developed and what caused it.

In the 1960s, with the new anatomical and chemical techniques, we could see the severe dopamine depletion in the corpus striatum (Ehringer & Hornykiewicz, 1960). The corpus striatum is in the middle of our brains, coordinating motor planning, decision-making, motivation, reinforcement, and reward perceptions. The 'shaking palsy' could now be classified as a dopamine deficiency disorder, and the various symptoms associated with the condition could be better understood.

Parkinson's symptoms come into two categories: motor and non-motor. Motor symptoms include freezing, rigidity, tremors, and difficulty moving. Non-motor symptoms include anxiety, depression, apathy, pain, fatigue, problems swallowing, and bowel and bladder difficulties. The symptoms vary a lot from person to person and have different impact on individual's lives. Of course, the symptoms might not be very severe, but that doesn't mean you are not frustrated having to deal with them. The symptoms you are experiencing are getting in the way of living the way you used to, the way you'd like to.

In the UK, 1 in 37 people will be diagnosed with Parkinson's in their lifetime, and men are 1.4 times more likely to be diagnosed than women (Parkinson's UK, 2024). However, the ratio is lower in Asia (0.95–1.2), possibly due to environmental and/or genetic factors. Interestingly, over the years, the incidence of Parkinson's in women has remained stable, whereas it has increased in men. Most people diagnosed with Parkinson's are over 50 years old, but 1 in 20 are under 40.

The incidence and prevalence of Parkinson's has increased rapidly throughout the world (Ou et al., 2021). Parkinson's might even be the fastest-growing neurological condition worldwide. The growth can be partly explained by the population's ageing because the incidence of Parkinson's increases with age. However, the rise in incidence is driven by more factors than ageing, such as the more accurate diagnostic process and environmental pollution with toxins. The larger the societal growth in gross national income, the faster the incidence of Parkinson's (Dorsey et al., 2018), perhaps because economic growth is a proxy for industrialisation and environmental pollution.

1.1 WHAT ARE THE POSSIBLE CAUSES AND RISK FACTORS OF PARKINSON'S?

When you got the diagnosis of Parkinson's, you might have wondered why that happened. Scientists have asked a similar question for years: What causes Parkinson's? While we don't know the exact cause, scientists have found some genetic and environmental factors are linked with the onset of Parkinson's and point to potential causes. We need to understand the possible triggers of Parkinson's to identify ways to prevent it and develop effective treatments.

In most populations, 3–5% of Parkinson's is explained by a single gene, whereas 90 genetic risk variants explain 16–36%. Although, in several studies, a positive family history has been associated with a high risk of Parkinson's, in most cases a clear mode of inheritance is difficult to establish (De Lau & Breteler, 2006). Still, a large percentage of cases are unexplained.

Knowledge of the genetic epidemiology of Parkinson's was advanced by conducting large-scale genome-wide association studies (Fung et al., 2006). A genome-wide association study is when researchers quickly scan for DNA variants in many individuals and check if it is associated with a trait or a disease. These studies confirmed the genes SNCA, PARK16, LRRK2, and MAPT as risk genes for Parkinson's (Verstraeten et al., 2015).

A head injury has been discussed as a trigger for Parkinson's and other neurological conditions. A head injury could cause neural inflammation, resulting in neurological changes we see in neurodegenerative conditions like Parkinson's (Smith et al., 2013). A 2018 study published in the *Neurology* journal looked at the health records of over 300,000 military veterans and found that for those with moderate brain injury (i.e. loss of consciousness for less than 30 minutes and memory loss for less than 24 hours), the risk for Parkinson's increased by 56% (Gardner et al., 2018). We also have some evidence suggesting that brain injury is associated with an onset of Parkinson's at an earlier age but not with more severe disease-associated nerve cell loss or younger age of death (Spiegel et al., 2021).

Although we see links between Parkinson's and brain injury, and there is a possible explanation for this relationship, we have mainly discovered this relationship by looking back at medical records. Someone with Parkinson's in an early stage of the condition with minimal symptoms has a higher risk of losing their balance and falling and suffering from a head injury compared with the general population.

Pesticide exposure and other environmental chemicals have also been related to the development of Parkinson's (Ascherio & Schwarzschild, 2016), and the evidence is substantial. However, still, we do not know much about specific compounds. Recently, the chemical trichloroethylene, which has been widely used in industrial cleaning products, has been reported to be associated with the development of Parkinson's. However, research in the area is emerging.

High dairy consumption has also been linked with an increased risk of Parkinson's (Ascherio & Schwarzschild, 2016), and this risk is more substantial in men than women (Jiang et al., 2014). More milk consumption was associated with decreased neuronal density in the substantia nigra, an effect we see in Parkinson's and especially in those who drank the most milk, as compared with those who did not drink milk (Abbott et al., 2016). There might be a possibility that a milk contaminant causes the problem and not the milk consumption. However, there are a lot of findings in different countries and, and the findings are consistent. A more probable explanation of the association between milk consumption and Parkinson's is that milk lowers uric acid, which we will see later as one of the protective factors against Parkinson's.

An increased risk of Parkinson's among individuals with melanoma is well documented. Recently, Zhang and colleagues gathered data from 63 studies that included over 17 million participants and found that people with Parkinson's had a 15% lower risk of developing cancer. Vice versa, individuals with cancer had a 26% lower risk of developing Parkinson's. These associations were the same whether we looked at smoking-related cancers and non-smoking related. In contrast, Parkinson's was associated with a 75% higher risk of melanoma (Zhang et al., 2021). Scientists explore various theories on why this association might exist. Hair/skin colour and genetic predisposition have been examined as potential culprits, but these theories have not been substantiated.

Let us move onto protective factors against Parkinson's. We have robust evidence on the role of uric acid as a protective factor. The body creates uric acid when it needs to break down purines. Purines are produced in the body and are also found in some foods, for example, liver, anchovies, mackerel, dried beans and peas, and beer. Most uric acid dissolves in blood and travels to the kidneys, passing out in urine. Scientists believe uric acid acts as an antioxidant, a feature that could potentially protect against what causes Parkinson's

(Ascherio & Schwarzschild, 2016). Moreover, uric acid levels are significantly lower in Parkinson's, which further decreases as the disease progresses (Wen et al., 2017).

Physical activity has also been found to be a protective factor against developing Parkinson's, as physical activity can have a neuroprotective effect, for example, by regulating dopamine. Interestingly, the protective effects of physical activity against Parkinson's seemed more significant for men and those engaging in moderate to vigorous exercise (Chen et al., 2021). However, Parkinson's has an insidious onset that precedes diagnosis by many years in the majority of cases, and people at this stage of the disease have a lower capacity for strenuous exercise. As a result, an individual, even before the diagnosis, is less likely to have increased physical activity than the general population (Ascherio & Schwarzschild, 2016).

Evidence suggests a protective effect of smoking on Parkinson's, that is, smoking lowers the risk of developing Parkinson's. Given the many harmful effects induced by tobacco, it was quite a paradox to observe a beneficial effect in the case of Parkinson's. An abundance of evidence supports this association, but conflict remains regarding its authenticity. Tobacco smoke comprises a variety of ingredients. Nicotine is believed to be responsible for the protective effect against Parkinson's. There is biological evidence to suggest that nicotine stimulates dopaminergic neurons and possesses a neuroprotective effect. However, the small studies in the area mean some of these effects might be biased and inflated. People with Parkinson's are less likely to be smokers, and smokers have a higher risk of death; therefore, smokers are underrepresented in Parkinson's.

Coffee and caffeine have also been identified as a protective factor in Parkinson's. Further, this is more true for men than women, probably because of an interaction between caffeine and postmenopausal hormones (Ascherio & Schwarzschild, 2016). Caffeine intake was associated with reduced Parkinson's disease risk among women not using postmenopausal hormones. There might be some interactions between caffeine and hormones that are not yet clear. Also, how much caffeine is associated with the protective effects is again unclear.

Anti-inflammatory drugs, especially ibuprofen, could also contribute to delaying or preventing the onset of Parkinson's and other neurodegenerative conditions by suppressing the pro-inflammatory responses. Ibuprofen use is associated with a 27% reduction in Parkinson's risk (Gao et al., 2011).

The causes of Parkinson's are not entirely clear, and likely, a combination of genetics, environmental exposures, and age-related changes in the brain contribute to its manifestation. The research evidence we have so far suggests that a collection of genes is responsible for Parkinson's in a small number of cases. Further, head injuries, pesticides, dairy consumption, and a history of melanoma might increase the risks of being diagnosed with Parkinson's. In contrast, caffeine consumption, physical activity, and use of ibuprofen might have a neuroprotective role.

1.2 WHAT ARE SOME COMMON EARLY AND LATER-ON PARKINSON'S SYMPTOMS?

In this section, I will be discussing many different symptoms related to Parkinson's. That doesn't mean you will experience them all. If reading about all potential symptoms of Parkinson's is upsetting and you'd rather not know, please skip this section, and move to another that might be more relevant and helpful to you.

Parkinson's does not announce itself all at once. Instead, it often creeps in gradually, showing up in ways that are easy to overlook until they begin to affect daily life. Early symptoms include constipation (the most common symptom), acting out dreams during the rapid eye movement (REM) phase of sleep, loss of smell, shoulder pain, mask-like facial expression, or depression (Armstrong & Okun, 2020). These early symptoms may also include tremors, stiffness, slow movement (bradykinesia), and impaired balance and coordination. The earliest stages of Parkinson's can be challenging to recognise, as reflected by the long delay (average ten years) that typically separates the person's first noticeable symptom from the timing of diagnosis (Gaenslen et al., 2011).

Parkinson's involves more than 30 motor symptoms and more than 40 non-motor symptoms. This chapter will explore the most common non-motor symptoms and how they can impact your daily life. While motor symptoms may dominate the narrative of Parkinson's, the non-motor symptoms often wield a profound impact on daily life (Santos García et al., 2019), and they do not commonly improve with dopaminergic medication (Kakkar & Dahiya, 2015; Rizek et al., 2016). In most cases, Parkinson's symptoms begin on one side of the body before affecting both sides over time.

Standard features include a stooped posture, limb and axial rigidity, and a shuffling gait with reduced arm swing. Bradykinesia (slowness of movement) can lead to an expressionless face (hypomimia) and progressively smaller handwriting (micrographia). Approximately 80% of individuals with Parkinson's experience limb tremors, most commonly a pill-rolling resting tremor of the hands. Tremors can also affect the legs and vary in presentation. Gait disturbances may include hesitation, freezing, and destination, where steps become smaller and faster, potentially leading to falls.

Freezing of movement occurs in 25–60% of individuals, typically several years after onset. Falls and postural instability may develop early or later in the disease course, with older age being a significant risk factor. Research has shown that over 60% of people with Parkinson's experience falls, often leading to hospital admissions (Sveinbjornsdottir, 2016).

Dystonia, uncontrolled and sometimes painful muscle movements, can appear before diagnosis or as a side effect of long-term treatment. It may affect the feet, hands, jaw, or neck and present as cramping, twisting, or rigidity. People with Parkinson's may develop changes in posture over time. Some individuals experience camptocormia, where the upper body bends forward, making it difficult to stand up straight. Others may have antercollis, where the head and neck tilt forward. Scoliosis, a sideways curve of the spine, can also occur. These changes are often caused by a combination of muscle stiffness (rigidity), involuntary muscle contractions (dystonia), muscle weakness, and difficulties sensing body position (impaired proprioception), making balance and movement more challenging.

Most common non-motor symptoms include mood (anxiety, depression, apathy – we will discuss these further in the following chapters), cognition, sleep disorders, gastrointestinal (swallowing, hypersalivation, constipation), hyperhidrosis, restless legs, sexual problems, delusions, and hallucinations.

Sleep problems are common, affecting around two-thirds of people with Parkinson's. This is due to changes in the brain structures and chemicals that regulate sleep, as well as the effects of Parkinson's medications. Many people with Parkinson's experience fragmented sleep, meaning they wake up frequently during the night. This can be caused by shallow sleep, difficulty turning in bed, frequent urination, nighttime tremors, and depression. Up to 50% of people with Parkinson's experience extreme tiredness during the day, which can be worsened by dopaminergic medications used to manage motor symptoms. Some individuals may also experience sudden sleep attacks, falling asleep without warning. Another common sleep disorder in Parkinson's is REM sleep behaviour disorder, where you physically act out your dreams by kicking, thrashing, or shouting in your sleep. This condition affects about 27–32% of people with Parkinson's and can appear years before other symptoms. Restless legs syndrome, a strong urge to move the legs when at rest, often relieved by walking, is another common symptom. Many people with Parkinson's also experience periodic leg movements of sleep, where the legs jerk involuntarily during sleep, and obstructive sleep apnoea. Some people with Parkinson's experience pauses in breathing while asleep, although research is mixed on whether this is more common in Parkinson's.

Hyperhidrosis (excessive sweating) is common in Parkinson's, and its frequency increases along with disease duration. Hyperhidrosis is associated not only with motor severity and motor complications such as dyskinesia (difficulties in movement) but also with non-motor symptoms such as sexual dysfunction and anxiety (Lin et al., 2022).

One of the most visible yet often misunderstood symptoms of Parkinson's is facial masking, a difficulty in expressing emotions through facial muscles, so people appear expressionless or unresponsive, even though they still experience emotions normally. You may smile less often or struggle to show expressions like surprise or anger. In addition, some individuals experience loss of prosody, the natural pitch and rhythm variations in speech that convey emotion, leading others to mistakenly perceive them as distant, uninterested, or emotionally detached. Studies suggest that difficulties in expressing emotions through facial expressions can also make it harder to recognise emotions in others, as mimicking expressions is essential to understanding them.

In addition to facial masking, other speech and communication challenges are also common in Parkinson's. Over 50% of people diagnosed with Parkinson's experience speech difficulties, such as quiet or hurried speech, while swallowing problems affect 40–80% and dribbling of saliva affects 25% of people (Sveinbjornsdottir, 2016). Dysarthria involves a monotone voice, reduced volume, and slurred or slowed speech. While medications like levodopa may help some aspects of speech, they often do not fully restore normal communication abilities. Fortunately, speech therapy and non-pharmacological interventions, such as facial exercises, voice training, and assistive communication devices, can improve expression and social confidence.

Digestive issues are common in Parkinson's due to the slowing of movement in the gastrointestinal tract. Many people experience bloating and delayed stomach emptying (gastric retention). The most frequent issue is constipation, affecting 70–80% of individuals with Parkinson's. Reduced physical activity, medication side effects, and changes in gut function can worsen this. Some people also have difficulty emptying the bowels due to problems with the rectal muscles.

Sexual difficulties are common in Parkinson's, affecting both men and women. In a study that included 100 people with Parkinson's, both the men and women reported frequent sexual problems before the diagnosis, and most of the men with sexual dysfunction were older than 60 years of age (85.5%) and living with their spouse (81.2%) (Bronner et al., 2023). Sexual function is a delicate balance of the mind and body, requiring seamless coordination between neurological, hormonal, vascular, and emotional systems. Parkinson's can disrupt this process. In a population of early-onset Parkinson's, it was found that factors like identifying as male, higher levels of depression, and higher urinary dysfunction were all related to reports of more sexual dysfunction (Vela-Desojo et al., 2020). Beyond the physical challenges, other psychosocial and personal factors also play a role. Relationship dynamics, cultural background, age, mood disorders, past experiences, disease stage, sleep disorders, and drug therapy can influence sexual well-being, both directly and indirectly (Meco et al., 2008).

Cognitive decline is common in Parkinson's and can occur at any stage, from mild difficulties to full dementia. Early symptoms often include challenges with planning, problem-solving, and organising tasks (executive function). Other issues, such as trouble with spatial awareness, slower speech, and memory difficulties, may also develop over time. Cognitive decline in Parkinson's is linked to the spread of brain changes affecting thinking and memory. Mild cognitive impairment is twice as common in people with Parkinson's compared to those without the disease. The risk of developing dementia increases with age and disease severity rather than the age at which Parkinson's starts. A six-year study following people with Parkinson's found that the risk of dementia increased from 8.5% in the first year to nearly 50% by year six (Pigott et al., 2015).

Many people with Parkinson's experience hallucinations and illusions, with visual hallucinations being the most common. Around 30–40% of individuals report seeing people, animals, or objects that are not there. These images may appear for seconds to minutes and often recur throughout the day. In most cases, people with Parkinson's retain insight and understand the hallucinations are not real. Although dopaminergic medications can trigger hallucinations, they can also occur before treatment begins, suggesting that Parkinson's-related changes in the brain, especially in the amygdala and hippocampus play a role. Other sensory hallucinations, such as smells, sounds, or physical sensations, are less common. In the later stages of Parkinson's, paranoia and delusions may develop, particularly in individuals with cognitive decline, depression, or advanced disease. This can lead to suspicion towards loved ones or beliefs that others are trying to cause harm.

Some people with Parkinson's may develop impulse control disorders due to dopaminergic medication, particularly dopamine agonists. This can lead to behaviours such as gambling, excessive spending, reckless decision-making, hypersexuality, or compulsive behaviours (e.g. hoarding), euphoria, overconfidence, or difficulty with planning and organisation. This condition, known as dopamine dysregulation syndrome, is more common in younger men with early-onset Parkinson's and is strongly linked to high doses of dopamine-based treatments.

Parkinson's affects men and women differently, not only in how it progresses but also in the symptoms they experience. Women with Parkinson's tend to report more mood disturbances, such as anxiety, depression, and apathy, along with greater fatigue, sleep problems, and pain. They also experience restless legs syndrome and facial masking more frequently than men. However, they tend to have a tremor-dominant form of Parkinson's, which often progresses more slowly, sometimes creating the false impression that their disease is milder. Women face a greater overall symptom burden, including a higher risk of dyskinesias (involuntary movements), non-motor fluctuations, and osteoporosis. These factors contribute to a greater impact on quality of life and increased feelings of stigma compared to men.

A small percentage of women, about 5%, are diagnosed with Parkinson's before the age of 40, a group known as young-onset Parkinson's disease. For these women, pregnancy, hormonal changes, and contraception choices become essential considerations. Some women notice a worsening of Parkinson's symptoms during pregnancy and the postpartum period, though the reasons for this are not yet well understood. There are no official guidelines on managing Parkinson's during pregnancy, and research on maternal safety, delivery options, postpartum depression, and foetal outcomes is limited. As we discussed earlier, the role of hormone replacement therapy is still not well understood in Parkinson's.

Beyond neurological symptoms, women with Parkinson's face additional health risks, including greater weight loss, and increased pelvic floor dysfunction compared to men. As a result, women with Parkinson's should receive early screening for osteoporosis, along with dietary guidance and physiotherapy to prevent bone deterioration and malnutrition. In addition, pelvic floor therapy can be beneficial in managing bladder and bowel symptoms that are more common in women.

Parkinson's is often thought of as a movement disorder. Still, it also includes an array of non-motor symptoms, like speech difficulties, sleep, mental health challenges, and issues with digestion and swallowing. Each symptom can affect you differently, but understanding them is the first step in managing them more effectively. In the following chapters, we'll focus on practical behavioural approaches, helping you build a personal plan to navigate life with Parkinson's.

1.3 WHAT TREATMENTS ARE AVAILABLE TO MANAGE THE SYMPTOMS AND SLOW THE PROGRESSION OF PARKINSON'S DISEASE?

Despite decades of progress in treating the symptoms of Parkinson's, the most pressing challenge remains: can we slow, stop, or reverse the progression of the disease itself? The desire for more than symptom relief, for a therapy that truly changes the course of Parkinson's is shared by everyone touched by the condition. Fortunately, research is beginning to move us closer to this goal. Two major approaches guide the search for disease-modifying therapies, treatments that not only ease symptoms but also intervene in the disease process.

The diagnostic criteria of Parkinson's include mostly motor symptoms that occur after loss of at least 50–60% of the nigral neurons. This damage is irreversible, and available treatment options do not alter it. Earlier diagnosis of the disease implies detecting the disease at a point with a small percentage of neuron loss. This could be the key to researching a disease-modifying treatment in a less advanced stage.

One line of research draws on epidemiological studies, which look at patterns in large populations. As we talked earlier, some studies have found that people who consume caffeine or nicotine have a lower risk of developing Parkinson's. While these substances are not cures, they have led scientists to explore whether certain common compounds might have protective effects on the brain. Caffeine, nicotine, and specific anti-inflammatory agents are now being studied for their potential to alter the disease course. These investigations could reveal ways to reduce risk or slow progression, particularly in people who are at higher genetic risk for Parkinson's.

The second, and perhaps more transformative, approach is based on breakthroughs in the genetic understanding of Parkinson's. Since the discovery of the first Parkinson's-related gene mutation (PARK1) in the late 1990s, research has focused on the abnormal protein alpha-synuclein, which plays a key role in Parkinson's. In people with the disease, this protein misfolds, clumps together, and spreads through the nervous system, damaging neurons. Pharmaceutical research is now aimed at interfering with this process by using antibodies to help the immune system clear out abnormal alpha-synuclein, stopping alpha-synuclein from aggregating in the first place, or enhancing natural processes like autophagy, which helps clear damaged proteins (Oertel, 2017).

One experimental treatment has attracted significant attention: nilotinib, a drug originally approved for treating leukaemia. In a small, early-stage study conducted at Georgetown University, 12 people with advanced Parkinson's, some of whom had cognitive decline, were given daily doses of nilotinib for six months (Pagan et al., 2016). To the surprise of many in the field, these people showed clinical improvements, sparking new hope. Animal studies have demonstrated that nilotinib could reduce alpha-synuclein accumulation and protect dopamine-producing neurons by enhancing autophagy. However, research evidence so far cannot confirm the clinical advantages of nilotinib (Xie et al., 2022).

Although these research developments are promising, there is still work to be done. Clinical trials must confirm safety, long-term effectiveness, and the ability to make a real difference in the lives of people with Parkinson's. Since there is no cure, current treatments focus on managing the symptoms, especially the movement-related ones. According to the National Institute for Health and Care Excellence (NICE, 2017), managing Parkinson's involves a wide range of professionals. Traditional management is focused on motor symptoms, and psychological support is limited and varies widely between regions.

A review of treatments for Parkinson's published in the *Neuroimmunology and Neuroinflammation* journal suggested that treatment approaches can vary and are often highly individualised (Lee & Yankee, 2021). They may include medication, physical and occupational therapy, surgical options like deep brain stimulation, or a combination of these. Deep brain stimulation is a surgical treatment that involves implanting electrodes into specific areas of the brain to regulate abnormal signals. Because Parkinson's is a progressive condition that affects people differently, treatments are adjusted over time to match changing needs and responses.

Most people with Parkinson's will be offered medication to help manage their motor symptoms. The most commonly used group of medications are dopaminergic drugs, medicines that either increase dopamine levels or mimic its effects on the brain. This is because many of the hallmark symptoms of Parkinson's, such as slowness of movement (bradykinesia), stiffness, and tremor, are linked to a reduction of dopamine in a part of the brain known as the nigrostriatal pathway (Lee & Yankee, 2021).

The most effective medication for treating these motor symptoms is levodopa (L-DOPA). This is considered the 'gold standard' for Parkinson's therapy. Levodopa works by crossing into the brain (where dopamine itself cannot go) and being converted into dopamine (Lee & Yankee, 2021). For many people, especially early in the disease, levodopa brings noticeable relief, especially in reducing stiffness and slowness. Another class of drugs, called dopamine agonists, acts directly on the brain's dopamine receptors, mimicking its effects. Depending on individual circumstances, these may be used alone or in combination with levodopa.

Not everyone responds the same way to Parkinson's medications. Around 80% of people with unknown cause Parkinson's (the most common form) respond well to levodopa, but the effectiveness of the drug can decline over time. It is also less effective for symptoms such as speech difficulties, balance problems, cognitive changes, and certain pain or sleep issues. Because of this, treatment decisions are made based on not only symptoms but also age, disease onset, lifestyle, and personal priorities. For example, in younger people with Parkinson's, doctors may delay starting levodopa to reduce the risk of developing dyskinesias, involuntary movements that can result from long-term use.

It is important to know that dyskinesia is not caused by levodopa alone. It appears to result from a combination of Parkinson's-related brain changes and the way levodopa is delivered in a *pulsed* (on-off) fashion. Newer ways of giving the drug, such as intestinal gel infusions, may reduce these effects in some people (Lee & Yankee, 2021).

Parkinson's symptoms evolve, and so must the treatment. People who begin on one medication may need to adjust doses or add new medications as the condition progresses. It is a process of careful monitoring and collaborative decision-making between the person with Parkinson's and their healthcare team.

For some people with Parkinson's, especially when medications no longer offer sufficient relief or cause problematic side effects, surgical options may be considered. These interventions aim to reduce symptoms, particularly motor difficulties like tremors, rigidity, and slowness of movement, but they do not stop the condition from progressing. There are three main types of surgical or investigational approaches used or studied for Parkinson's: ablative surgery, deep brain stimulation, and cell or gene-based therapies.

Ablative surgery is the oldest form of surgical treatment for Parkinson's. It involves creating a small, targeted lesion (or area of damage) in specific regions of the brain that are overactive in Parkinson's. By disrupting these abnormal signals, the aim is to improve motor symptoms. There are three primary forms: pallidotomy (targeting the globus pallidus), thalamotomy (targeting the thalamus), and subthalamotomy (targeting the subthalamic nucleus) (Lee & Yankee, 2021). However, complications such as vision changes, speech issues, and weakness can occur, especially with procedures performed on both sides of the brain. Because of the potential risks, ablative surgery is now less common. However, it can still be a viable treatment in some instances, particularly where other options like deep brain stimulation are unavailable or unsuitable.

Deep brain stimulation has become one of the most commonly used surgical treatments for Parkinson's. Deep brain stimulation, rather than destroying brain tissue, uses small electrical impulses to regulate abnormal brain activity.

A small device, like a pacemaker, is implanted under the skin of the chest and connected by wires to electrodes placed in specific brain regions (commonly the subthalamic nucleus or the globus pallidus interna). Deep brain stimulation can help reduce tremors and rigidity, minimise 'off' periods (when medication is not working well) and potentially lower the need for Parkinson's drugs, particularly after stimulation of the subthalamic nucleus.

However, not all symptoms respond equally. Problems like speech changes, balance difficulties, and cognitive changes may not improve, and, in some cases, may worsen. Side effects can include slurred speech, dizziness, or involuntary movements. While deep brain stimulation is well established and has helped many people, researchers are exploring newer forms, like 'closed-loop deep brain stimulation', which adapts real-time stimulation based on the brain's activity. This may lead to fewer side effects and better, more personalised results.

As the understanding of Parkinson's deepens, new frontiers in treatment are being explored, particularly cell transplantation and gene therapy. Cell transplantation involves replacing damaged or lost dopamine-producing cells in the brain with healthy ones, often using foetal cells, embryonic stem cells, or induced pluripotent stem cells. Early research has shown that transplanted cells can survive, grow, and connect with existing brain circuits in animal models. Though still experimental, this therapy offers hope that one day, we may be able to restore the brain's natural ability to produce dopamine.

Gene therapy aims to deliver new genetic instructions to the brain to help the brain make more dopamine or protect it from further damage. Some approaches try to increase the levels of key enzymes involved in dopamine production, potentially making current medications more effective or reducing the dose needed. Gene therapy is still in clinical trials, but early results show promise for helping with motor symptoms. It cannot yet treat non-motor symptoms like mood or sleep disturbances, but it is a fast-evolving field with exciting potential.

Research is beginning to move us closer to finding a cure for Parkinson's. Various disease-modifying therapies that could intervene in the disease process itself are investigated. However, these treatments are still in the experimental phases. However, we have a range of pharmacological treatments, brain stimulations, and non-pharmacological therapies that can help manage symptoms and improve the overall quality of life.

FURTHER READING

Here are some links to websites that expand on what we know about Parkinson's if you would like to find out more.

Cure Parkinson's. (n.d.). *About Parkinson's*. Retrieved June 4, 2025, from https://cureparkinsons.org.uk/about-parkinsons/

Lee, T. K., & Yankee, E. L. (2021). A review on Parkinson's disease treatment. *Neuroimmunology and Neuroinflammation*, *8*.

Parkinson's Foundation. (n.d.). *Understanding Parkinson's*. Retrieved June 4, 2025, from https://www.parkinson.org/understanding-parkinsons

Parkinson's UK. (n.d.). *Newly diagnosed with Parkinson's*. Retrieved June 4, 2025, from https://www.parkinsons.org.uk/information-and-support/newly-diagnosed-parkinsons

REFERENCES

Abbott, R. D., Ross, G. W., Petrovitch, H., Masaki, K. H., Launer, L. J., Nelson, J. S., White, L. R., & Tanner, C. M. (2016). Midlife milk consumption and substantia nigra neuron density at death. *Neurology*, *86*(6), 512–519.

Armstrong, M. J., & Okun, M. S. (2020). Diagnosis and treatment of Parkinson disease: A review. *JAMA*, *323*, 548–560.

Ascherio, A., & Schwarzschild, M. A. (2016). The epidemiology of Parkinson's disease: Risk factors and prevention. *The Lancet Neurology*, *15*(12), 1257–1272.

Bronner, G., Peleg-Nesher, S., Manor, Y., Rosenberg, A., Naor, S., Taichman, T., Ezra, A., & Gurevich, T. (2023). Sexual needs and sexual function of patients with Parkinson's disease. *Neurological Sciences*, *44*(2), 539–546.

Chen, Y., Sun, X., Lin, Y., Zhang, Z., Gao, Y., & Wu, I. X. (2021). Non-genetic risk factors for Parkinson's disease: An overview of 46 systematic reviews. *Journal of Parkinson's Disease*, *11*(3), 919–935.

De Lau, L. M., & Breteler, M. M. (2006). Epidemiology of Parkinson's disease. *The Lancet Neurology*, *5*(6), 525–535.

Dorsey, E. R., Sherer, T., Okun, M. S., & Bloem, B. R. (2018). The emerging evidence of the Parkinson pandemic. *Journal of Parkinson's Disease*, *8*, S3–S8.

Ehringer, H., & Hornykiewicz, O. (1960). Verteilung von Noradrenalin und Dopamin (3-Hy[1]droxytyramin) im Gehirn des Menschen und ihr Verhalten bei Erkrankungen des ex[1]trapyramidalen Systems. *Klin Wochenschr*, *38*, 1236–1239.

Fung, H. C., Scholz, S., Matarin, M., Simón-Sánchez, J., Hernandez, D., Britton, A., Gibbs, J. R., Langefeld, C., Stiegert, M. L., Schymick, J., Okun,

M. S., Mandel, R. J., Fernandez, H. H., Foote, K. D., Rodríguez, R., Peckham, E., De Vrieze, F. W., Gwinn-Hardy, K., Hardy, J. A., & Singleton, A. (2006). Genome-wide genotyping in Parkinson's disease and neurologically normal controls: First stage analysis and public release of data. *The Lancet Neurology*, *5*(11), 911–916.

Gaenslen, A., Swid, I., Liepelt-Scarfone, I., Godau, J., & Berg, D. (2011). The patients' perception of prodromal symptoms before the initial diagnosis of Parkinson's disease. *Movement Disorders*, *26*, 653–658.

Gao, X., Chen, H., Schwarzschild, M. A., & Ascherio, A. (2011). Use of ibuprofen and risk of Parkinson disease. *Neurology*, *76*(10), 863–869.

Gardner, R. C., Byers, A. L., Barnes, D. E., Li, Y., Boscardin, J., & Yaffe, K. (2018). Mild TBI and risk of Parkinson disease: A chronic effects of neurotrauma consortium study. *Neurology*, *90*(20), e1771–e1779.

Jiang, W., Ju, C., Jiang, H., & Zhang, D. (2014). Dairy foods intake and risk of Parkinson's disease: A dose–response meta-analysis of prospective cohort studies. *European Journal of Epidemiology*, *29*(9), 613–619.

Kakkar, A. K., & Dahiya, N. (2015). Management of Parkinson's disease: Current and future pharmacotherapy. *European Journal of Pharmacology*, *750*, 74–81.

Lee, T. K., & Yankee, E. L. (2021). A review on Parkinson's disease treatment. *Neuroimmunology and Neuroinflammation*, *8*.

Lees, A. J., Ferreira, J., Rascol, O., Poewe, W., Rocha, J. F., McCrory, M., Soares-da-Silva, P., & BIPARK-2 Study Investigators. (2017). Opicapone as adjunct to levodopa therapy in patients with Parkinson disease and motor fluctuations: A randomized clinical trial. *JAMA Neurology*, *74*(2), 197–206.

Lin, J., Ou, R., Wei, Q., Cao, B., Li, C., Hou, Y., Zhang, L., Liu, K., & Shang, H. (2022). Hyperhidrosis in Parkinson's disease: A 3-year prospective cohort study. *Journal of the European Academy of Dermatology and Venereology*, *36*(7), 1104–1112.

Meco, G., Rubino, A., Caravona, N., & Valente, M. (2008). Sexual dysfunction in Parkinson's disease. *Parkinsonism & Related Disorders*, *14*(6), 451–456.

National Institute for Health and Care Excellence (Great Britain). (2017). *Parkinson's disease in adults: Diagnosis and management: Full guideline.* National Institute for Health and Care Excellence.

Oertel, W. H. (2017). Recent advances in treating Parkinson's disease. *F1000Research*, *6*, 260.

Ou, Z., Pan, J., Tang, S., Duan, D., Yu, D., Nong, H., & Wang, Z. (2021). Global trends in the incidence, prevalence, and years lived with disability of Parkinson's disease in 204 countries/territories from 1990 to 2019. *Frontiers in Public Health*, *9*, 776847.

Pagan, F., Hebron, M., Valadez, E. H., Torres-Yaghi, Y., Huang, X., Mills, R. R., Wilmarth, B. M., Howard, H., Dunn, C., Carlson, A., Lawler, A., Rogers, S. L., Falconer, R. A., Ahn, J., Li, Z., & Moussa, C. (2016). Nilotinib effects in Parkinson's disease and dementia with Lewy bodies. *Journal of Parkinson's Disease*, *6*(3), 503–517.

Parkinson, J. (1817). *An essay on the shaking palsy*. Whittingham and Rowland for Sherwood, Needly and Jones.

Parkinson's UK. (2017). *The incidence and prevalence of Parkinson's in the UK: Results from the clinical practice research datalink summary report*. Retrieved June 2024, from https://www.parkinsons.org.uk/sites/default/files/2018-01/CS2960%20Incidence%20and%20prevalence%20report%20branding%20summary%20report%20Published%202017.pdf

Pigott, K., Rick, J., Xie, S. X., Hurtig, H., Chen-Plotkin, A., Duda, J. E., Morley, J. F., Chahine, L. M., Dahodwala, N., Akhtar, R. S., Siderowf, A., Trojanowski, J. Q., & Weintraub, D. (2015). Longitudinal study of normal cognition in Parkinson's disease. *Neurology*, *85*, 1276–1282.

Rizek, P., Kumar, N., & Jog, M. S. (2016). An update on the diagnosis and treatment of Parkinson disease. *Canadian Medical Association Journal*, *188*(16), 1157–1165.

Santos García, D., de Deus Fonticoba, T., Suárez Castro, E., Borrué, C., Mata, M., Solano Vila, B., Cots Foraster, A., Álvarez Sauco, M., Rodríguez Pérez, A. B., Vela, L., Macías, Y., Escalante, S., Esteve, P., Reverté Villarroya, S., Cubo, E., Casas, E., Arnaiz, S., Carrillo Padilla, F., Pueyo Morlans, M., . . . COPPADIS Study Group. (2019). Non-motor symptoms burden, mood, and gait problems are the most significant factors contributing to a poor quality of life in non-demented Parkinson's disease patients: Results from the COPPADIS Study Cohort. *Parkinsonism & Related Disorders*, *66*, 151–157.

Smith, C., Gentleman, S. M., Leclercq, P. D., Murray, L. S., Griffin, W. S. T., Graham, D. I., & Nicoll, J. A. (2013). The neuroinflammatory response in humans after traumatic brain injury. *Neuropathology and Applied Neurobiology*, *39*(6), 654–666.

Spiegel, J., Sone, J. Y., Butler, T., Pirraglia, E., & de Leon, M. J. (2021). Traumatic brain injury accelerates Parkinson's disease onset without altering Parkinson's neuropathology. *Alzheimer's & Dementia, 17*, e051517.

Sveinbjornsdottir, S. (2016). The clinical symptoms of Parkinson's disease. *Journal of Neurochemistry, 139*, 318–324.

Vela-Desojo, L., Urso, D., Kurtis-Urra, M., García-Ruiz, P. J., Pérez-Fernández, E., Lopez-Valdes, E., Posada-Rodriguez, I., Ybot-Gorrin, I., Lopez-Manzanares, L., Mata, M., Borrue, C., Ruiz-Huete, C., Maria Del Valle, M., & Martinez-Castrillo, J. C. (2020). Sexual dysfunction in early-onset Parkinson's disease: A cross-sectional, multicenter study. *Journal of Parkinson's Disease, 10*(4), 1621–1629.

Verstraeten, A., Theuns, J., & Van Broeckhoven, C. (2015). Progress in unraveling the genetic etiology of Parkinson disease in a genomic era. *Trends in Genetics, 31*(3), 140–149.

Wen, M., Zhou, B., Chen, Y. H., Ma, Z. L., Gou, Y., Zhang, C. L., Yu, W. F., & Jiao, L. (2017). Serum uric acid levels in patients with Parkinson's disease: A meta-analysis. *PLOS One, 12*(3), e0173731.

Xie, X., Yuan, P., Kou, L., Chen, X., Li, J., & Li, Y. (2022). Nilotinib in Parkinson's disease: A systematic review and meta-analysis. *Frontiers in Aging Neuroscience, 14*, 996217.

Zhang, X., Guarin, D., Mohammadzadeh Honarvar, N., Chen, X., & Gao, X. (2021). Parkinson's disease and cancer: A systematic review and meta-analysis of over 17 million participants. *BMJ Open, 11*(7), e046329.

2

WHAT PSYCHOLOGICAL SKILLS CAN HELP ME MANAGE PARKINSON'S CHALLENGES?

If you are still not able to process and accept the diagnosis of Parkinson's. If you feel like Parkinson's gets in the way of your plans and life. If you feel annoyed, angry, anxious, and fearful of the future frequently, sometimes multiple times a day. You are not alone, and maybe this section can provide some reassurance and help.

Everyone will have their response and way of dealing with a potentially life-changing diagnosis. There is no right way to act. You may feel relieved that you finally have a name to put to the cause of your symptoms. If you suspected you had Parkinson's, you may feel a sense of closure. Alongside these feelings, though, a Parkinson's diagnosis can still be potentially devastating and leave you in a state of shock.

Humans need emotions to survive; they are responses to external situations and internal thoughts and dialogues. Emotions keep us safe, prompt us into action, or hold us back from impulsive action; emotions help us survive and become and remain part of society; we are social animals, after all, and we need to be accepted by our tribe. If we were not anxious about the future, we would not be prompted to plan and organise things to avoid future threats; if we did not feel disgust, we would consume dangerous substances for survival.

DOI: 10.4324/9781003484332-3

Research has shown that about 22% of people with Parkinson's experience minor depression, 13% dysthymia (a mild form of depression), and roughly 17% meet the criteria for major depressive disorder (Reijnders et al., 2008). Depression could be an early symptom of Parkinson's. Some studies suggest that individuals diagnosed with Parkinson's were more likely to have been diagnosed with depression shortly before their Parkinson's diagnosis (Aarsland et al., 2012; Jacob et al., 2010). On a neurobiological level, depression in Parkinson's is linked to changes in key brain systems, including dopaminergic, noradrenergic, and serotoninergic pathways, with disruptions in neurotransmitter signalling, structural brain alterations, and shifts in inflammatory factors all contributing to the emotional impact (Aarsland et al., 2012).

Apart from the neurobiological changes linked to Parkinson's that can cause anxiety and depressive symptoms, you also have the emotional response to dealing with the initial diagnosis. It is natural to need time to come to terms with the diagnosis. Being diagnosed with a long-term condition has been compared to experiencing grief after a loss. There are different emotional stages to work through. There is no set time for working through this process – it will be different for everybody. But working through this grief you can reach a better place.

In the early stages, individuals grapple with what the diagnosis means for their identity, acknowledging how ongoing deterioration might limit their ability to engage in valued roles and activities. In a 2022 paper published in *Disability and Rehabilitation*, researchers examined 21 individual interview-based research studies to better understand people's experiences with a Parkinson's diagnosis. The common theme across all the studies was that for many, receiving a Parkinson's diagnosis is a transformative and deeply emotional experience (Wieringa et al., 2022).

Uncertainty can be one of the most challenging aspects of a Parkinson's diagnosis. The more you understand Parkinson's, the better equipped you will be to make informed decisions about your health and future. You can list questions or concerns and discuss them with your Parkinson's nurse, GP, or Parkinson's specialist. Perhaps, join a local Parkinson's support group or connect with national charities that provide reliable information and resources. And remember, no question is too small or unimportant; getting the right information can ease anxiety and help you take proactive steps.

We have a natural tendency to worry about things that are out of our control. However, this can lead to a great deal of fear and concern about the future. While acknowledging and accepting that the future is uncertain is important, it can also be helpful to adjust your thinking. Try looking at things from a different perspective by asking yourself: What *can* I control right now?

This can help you to feel more grounded. There are many aspects of your health that *are* still in your control. You can explore treatments that can help manage your symptoms – these options can reduce the impact your symptoms are having on your daily life, pharmacological treatment options include those discussed in the previous chapter, and non-pharmacological treatments are discussed in Chapter 4. Some people also find it empowering when keeping up to date with the latest Parkinson's research or by getting involved in clinical trials.

Receiving a Parkinson's diagnosis can be overwhelming, but there are ways to navigate this new reality and regain a sense of control. Seeking help soon after the diagnosis might support you with regaining a sense of control. A survey by Parkinson's UK showed that mental health was a significant challenge, especially for those in the first couple of years of their diagnosis (Deane et al., 2014). Talking therapies can provide valuable tools to help you process your emotions, build resilience, and develop practical coping strategies. Cognitive behavioural therapy can help reframe unhelpful thoughts and manage anxiety or low mood. Acceptance and commitment therapy focuses on embracing change, and living a fulfilling life despite challenges. Talk to your Parkinson's nurse or GP about a referral to a talking therapy service. In many areas, you can also self-refer to talking therapy services through the National Health Services website. Professional support can help you feel more in control and provide guidance tailored to your needs.

Talking therapies are now frequently delivered over the phone or online, which make them more convenient and accessible, while retaining their effectiveness. Two randomised controlled trials of a telemedicine intervention found that a three-month course of cognitive behavioural therapy tailored for Parkinson's (administered either by phone or web-based video conferencing) was associated with statistically and clinically significant improvements in depression compared with usual care (Dobkin et al., 2018, 2020) with results equivalent to those previously observed in face-to-face trials.

Let's look at two examples.

> Psychological therapies will not change your symptoms, but will change how much they affect your life. Ali experiences severe Parkinson's symptoms. He is in pain most of the time and can't sleep. He took early retirement and now at 55, he spends his days sitting at home bored. He avoids most physical activity because of the pain, and rigidity. He has become very irritable. Most people, including his family, don't enjoy his company. It even seems too much trouble when the grandchildren he adores come to visit.
>
> Isla, age 66, also experience severe Parkinson's symptoms. Everyday she manages to walk half a kilometer to the local library or the park. When the pain is severe, she practices relaxation techniques or tries to distract herself. She works a few hours a week as a volunteer at a local hospital. She also loves going to see her young grandchildren and even manages to take care of them for short periods of time. Her husband is amazed at how much zest she has for life.

Ali and Isla both live with the same condition with similar physical problems. Yet, their ability to function and enjoy life is very different. Why? The difference lies on factors we cannot see. For example, whether they also experience mental health challenges that are unaddressed, the severity of their symptoms, their support network, and also on their response to physical symptoms they are experiencing. Ali's life seems to have withered, whereas Isla has retained her previous sense of self by identifying other relevant activities that align with her core identity. Even though she has limitations, she controls her life instead of letting the condition control her.

Your response cannot change Parkinson's and prevent physical, cognitive, and psychological symptoms from developing, but a proactive (not re-active) response and certain self-management skills can make it much easier to live with. Much research now shows that the experience of pain discomfort and disability can be modified by circumstances, beliefs, mood, and the attention we pay to symptoms. What goes on in a person's mind is at least as important as what is going on in the person's body.

You might find it helpful to talk about the changes, any sense of loss, or the impact of your feelings with someone you trust. It is natural to feel like you do not want to 'burden' loved ones with your worries, but the truth is, they want to be there for you. Opening up about your feelings can strengthen your relationships and provide much-needed emotional relief. Talk to your family and friends about what you're experiencing. More often than not, they will be relieved you are sharing rather than bottling things up.

Sometimes, it helps to talk to people who truly understand what you're going through. Support groups, whether in-person or online, can provide a safe space to share experiences, exchange tips, and find encouragement. Some people enjoy the social aspect of local meetings, while others prefer the privacy and flexibility of online forums. Find what works best for you. Peer support can be empowering, helping you see that you're not alone in this journey. Many groups also invite guest speakers, such as medical professionals or therapists, who can provide valuable insights and advice.

In the following chapters we will explore steps to look after your body. For instance, working on your fitness and activity levels so your body is best prepared to face any challenges Parkinson's may bring. Looking after your brain and emotional health can also help with feeling in control. You can keep your brain healthy by exercising regularly, maintaining a healthy weight, reducing alcohol, and avoiding smoking. Keep your mind active through reading, puzzles, and creative activities (like painting, doing crafts, learning a language, and playing an instrument). Making time for the things you enjoy, scheduling some self-care time, and practise mindfulness and relaxation techniques can help. It may also help to learn more about your condition, become an expert on your Parkinson's and what's normal for you. That way, if anything changes you can be proactive and discuss things with your medical team early. And, of course, follow your treatment plan, this will ensure your Parkinson's symptoms are being managed as well as possible, and your Parkinson's is kept under control.

Having a plan for if your symptoms worsen can provide some reassurance/peace of mind, as you know what the next steps are if your situation changes. Thinking about the future can feel daunting, but having a plan in place can bring peace of mind. Advance care planning allows you to explore future care options and make your wishes known, so you and your loved ones feel prepared. Consider discussing your preferences for medical treatment, daily care, and quality of life with your family and healthcare team. Also, record important decisions so that if challenges arise, your loved ones and medical professionals will know how best to support you. Planning doesn't mean giving up hope. It is about ensuring that your needs and wishes are respected, allowing you to focus on living well today.

2.1 WHAT PSYCHOLOGICAL SKILLS CAN HELP ME MANAGE PARKINSON'S CHALLENGES?

Mental health in Parkinson's is often misunderstood, overlooked, or mistaken for something else. Apathy is dismissed as laziness, anxiety as mere worry, depression as a natural response to illness. But what if these emotional changes are not just reactions to Parkinson's, what if they are *part* of it, woven into the very fabric of the condition? Historically, our understanding of psychological difficulties in Parkinson's has been dominated by neurobiological explanations, such as changes in dopaminergic systems (Chaudhuri & Schapira, 2009). More recently, however, it has been recognised that psychological difficulties in Parkinson's are likely caused by a combination of neurobiological and psychological factors (Simpson et al., 2013; Weintraub & Burn, 2011).

Psychological difficulties are not just internally generated (i.e. via thinking unhelpful thoughts) or the product of biochemical changes. There are also harmful psychological effects of living in a culture which views disability as an individual construct rather than as a result of an ill-equipped society which is sometimes poorly motivated to accommodate fully all those with long-term conditions (Simpson & Thomas, 2015). Beyond motor and non-motor symptoms, people with Parkinson's also experience a negative emotional impact from society's attitudes and social interactions. For example, people living with Parkinson's can experience hurtful comments from others, being stared at, or being treated as less capable, and these social experiences can damage self-esteem and make people withdraw from social life. There are also other structural barriers, for example, feeling excluded from spaces or facing workplace discrimination can also lead to frustration, anxiety, and depression.

Social factors that contribute to the experiences of emotional difficulties are not frequently acknowledged. Many challenges faced by people with Parkinson's are not due to the condition itself but to a world that fails to accommodate their needs. This is known as structural disablism, when environments, policies, and societal norms make life more difficult. For example, buildings and public spaces that are inaccessible or difficult to navigate, workplace discrimination or forced early retirement due to employers' reluctance to provide accommodations, financial strain from the costs of care, home modifications, and lost income, as well as limited access to information and services in Parkinson's-friendly formats.

Studies show that nearly half of people with Parkinson's of working age are forced to stop working within five years of diagnosis. This loss of employment does not just impact finances, it affects independence, self-worth, and social identity, all of which can lead to emotional distress.

One of the most damaging effects of these experiences is internalised stigma, when a person starts believing negative stereotypes about their own condition. This can lead to self-imposed restrictions, such as avoiding social situations or not asking for help when needed. The way Parkinson's is perceived and accommodated in society affects mental health just as much as the disease itself. Feelings of isolation, frustration, and financial stress can increase anxiety and depression, making it even harder to manage Parkinson's symptoms.

Even though, in this chapter I will focus on the individual strategies you can implement to manage Parkinson's symptoms, I am deeply aware that there is also a societal responsibility and a shift that needs to happen at a higher level to accommodate and help individuals to live well with a long-term condition.

Before we delve into strategies, let's have a quick look at the importance of mental health for your quality of life and overall health, why and how it is developed and how common it is in Parkinson's.

Feeling frustrated, angry, or sad is very common and usual emotional response to the daily challenges of Parkinson's. It might be difficult at times to keep a positive attitude, especially when you feel unwell and your future appears uncertain. Feeling low and at a loss is normal and to be expected. Although small levels of distress can push us into action and motivate changes, being significantly depressed or anxious might have an adverse impact on the prognosis of the condition or even worsen the symptoms. A large study published on *Movement Disorders* looked at various motor and non-motor symptoms and the impact they had on 462 people with Parkinson's health status. The study showed that depression has more than twice the impact on health status compared to motor symptoms. Anxiety and other non-motor symptoms are also important separate factors that impact poor health status in Parkinson's (Hinnell et al., 2012). A smaller but more recent study has also showed similar results of the effects of both motor and non-motor symptoms on health-related quality of life (Candel-Parra et al., 2022).

Psychological distress can occur at any time throughout the course of Parkinson's. This may include mood challenges prior to diagnosis; psychological reactions to the initial diagnosis, and changes experienced as the condition progresses; psychological challenges caused by changes in neurotransmitter, inflammatory, and neurotrophic factors; and the psychological side-effects of dopaminergic treatment (Even & Weintraub, 2012).

The link of Parkinson's with depression gets even more complicated as the two conditions have similar symptoms, which makes a diagnosis challenging. Frequently depression is a symptom observed before the diagnosis of Parkinson's (Ishihara & Brayne, 2006). Depressive symptoms are common in Parkinson's and influence many other clinical aspects of the disease. You might be feeling worried or sad about things you can no longer do due to Parkinson's but clinical depression is more about not feeling enjoyment doing the things you used to find enjoyable. Clinical depression is characterised by excessive worrying, persistent sadness, crying, loss of interest in usual activities and hobbies, increased fatigue and lack of energy, feelings of guilt, loss of motivation, complaints of aches and pains, feelings of being a burden to loved ones and ruminations about disability, death and dying. If these symptoms feel familiar, it is a good idea to discuss them further with your doctor. People who experience more uncontrolled 'on–off' periods and freezing episodes are more prone to also experience depression. Further, poor sleep, constipation, and fatigue, can make depression symptoms worse, which is why it is important to take care of these factors as we will see in the following chapters.

Treatment mainly includes anti-depressive medications and behavioural interventions as psychotherapy. Psychological interventions, like group cognitive therapy, can improve mood and lessen depression (Yazd et al., 2023). Also, doing activities like exercises; having some sort of social interaction (e.g. meeting a friend for coffee, calling a relative, or stopping to talk to a neighbour while you take your daily walk), hobbies, or other activities that bring joy, comfort, and peace (e.g. listening to your favourite piece of music, taking a warm bath, meditating, or watching a movie); and eating well can all help boost mood.

Anxiety is also common but under-recognised, affecting approximately 31% of people with Parkinson's. Like depression, it often appears before motor symptoms, sometimes by two decades, and can persist throughout the disease. The most frequently diagnosed anxiety disorders in Parkinson's include generalised anxiety disorder (14%), social anxiety (13.8%), and panic disorder (6.8%), while a significant number of people experience multiple anxiety disorders at once. Anxiety adds to the complexity of Parkinson's, lowering individuals' quality of life (Dissanayaka et al., 2010).

The clinical characteristics of anxiety include avoidance, apprehension, worrying, anticipation, overly detailed, emotional reactivity, fearfulness, concerns about your health, and rumination – all these can lead to very real physical symptoms. In people with Parkinson's, this can mean the racing heart and trouble breathing of a panic attack, but it can also mean reduced motor function, such as impaired gait.

Feeling worry, uneasiness, guilt, and stress can be a normal part of life and can be resolved with time. However, clinical anxiety is more severe, persists for a long period, and interferes with daily activities. When this happens, anxiety is considered a disorder for which treatment is recommended. People with Parkinson's also sometimes feel anxious before they get their next dose of dopaminergic medication, as their symptoms begin to increase. Keep a log and tell your doctor or nurse when you experience increased anxiousness, so they can help you manage 'off'-state anxiety.

Many factors contribute to cause anxiety in Parkinson's, involving a mix of neurological, psychological, and social factors. Changes in dopamine, serotonin, and noradrenaline systems are believed to contribute to anxiety, along with alterations in key brain regions like the amygdala and cingulate cortex, which regulate fear and emotional processing. Anxiety does not cause illness progression, but when people progress, they feel more anxious. However, unlike motor symptoms, anxiety does not always improve with dopamine treatment, suggesting other neurochemical factors are at play. People with pessimistic or avoidant personality traits are more likely to develop anxiety, likely due to difficulty coping with the uncertainties of the disease. In contrast, those with strong social support networks and a clear sense of identity tend to experience less anxiety. Interestingly, research has shown that when people believe that the cause of their Parkinson's was due to a psychosocial cause, stress, overwork, and family and emotional difficulties, they tended to also experience higher anxiety. In other words, the higher anxiety that was experienced prior to the diagnosis, and which people believed caused the condition, could also extend after the diagnosis (Simpson et al., 2013).

Anxiety directly impacts quality of life, daily functioning, and even disease progression. People with Parkinson's and anxiety often experience increased sleep disturbances, greater difficulty with movement and mobility, higher risk of depression and reduced ability to participate in social and daily activities.

Apathy is another common mental health symptom of Parkinson's. Apathy affects motivation, emotions, and cognitive engagement and it is associated with reduced ability to carry out daily activities, lower response to treatment, poorer overall health outcomes, and quality of life. Apathy is characterised by a loss of interest and pleasure (anhedonia), an overlapping symptom with depression; however, unlike simple depression, apathy manifests as a persistent lack of goal-directed behaviour, reduced interest in activities, difficulty initiating or maintaining interest in mental activities, a struggle to self-motivate or initiate tasks, and diminished emotional response, without being caused by cognitive decline or emotional distress. Apathy tends to be more common in older individuals, and it has been linked to worse motor symptoms, greater executive dysfunction, and an increased risk of developing dementia.

People with Parkinson's describe apathy as reduced motivation due to the consequences and impairment of the condition, as creeping into jobs that they used to be able to do and no longer can do. People also talk about the (un)acceptability of apathy, the feeling that they have to complete certain number of tasks at the end of the day and also people discuss how others and the society expects them to do things, complete tasks and if not, that's frowned upon (Simpson et al., 2014).

As with other mental health issues, apathy can appear before the first noticeable motor symptoms. Depending on how it is diagnosed, studies suggest that between 20% and 36% of newly diagnosed people experience apathy before starting their treatment. In the early stages of Parkinson's, apathy often improves when the dopaminergic treatment works optimally, but as the disease progresses, it becomes more common again. Behavioural interventions can help with apathy, for example, setting concrete and obtainable goals or an activity list to follow through. Also, dance and music therapy, exercise, crafts, outings, and cognitive challenges like computer games, card games, puzzles, could help.

Apathy could be mistaken for depression but the two psychological challenges are different and it is important to disentangle the two as the medication used for depression will not improve apathy, even though, you could experience both (Den Brok et al., 2015). Depression is characterised by sadness, being worried and feeling hopeless, whereas apathy is the inability to 'get up and go'.

Apathy in Parkinson's disease is more likely to be a direct consequence of disease-related physiological changes than a psychological reaction or adaptation to disability and it is closely associated with cognitive impairment. These findings point to a possible role of cognitive mechanisms in the expression of apathy (Pluck & Brown, 2002).

Mental health issues are common in Parkinson's, but unfortunately, they are frequently overlooked. In a lot of cases mental health symptoms, especially anxiety and depression will appear before motor symptoms and before the diagnosis. Mental health difficulties have been found to be linked with lower quality of life and lower overall health status. So, what can be done? Pharmacological treatments have been found effective as well as cognitive behaviour therapy. Treating mental health as any other physical symptom of Parkinson's will help you appropriately manage it. There are also things you could do to help with cultivating resilience and learn coping things that can help you with everyday challenges and frustrations.

Given the multiple physical symptoms experienced by individuals with Parkinson's, it is likely that psychological interventions might also work best when physical symptoms are optimally controlled and vice versa. Over-identifying with the condition, arranging all your life around it and when Parkinson's occupy a large amount of your thoughts and energy creates more emotional distress. On the other hand, not engaging with the condition, not understanding it, and not adhering to the treatment can also result in increased distress. There is a delicate balance between the two extremes that can help you lead a rich and meaningful life while looking after your health and managing symptoms when needed.

2.2 HOW CAN I MANAGE FEELING STRESSED, FRUSTRATED, AND SAD?

You picked up this book which means you have either been diagnosed recently. You do not know where to start fitting Parkinson's in your life or you had Parkinson's for some time and have found some tricks that work for you but you want to know more about how to build a full and meaningful life and not just tick boxes of the things you need to do in relation to Parkinson's.

Maybe you think that experiencing anxiety and admitting it is like admitting you cannot cope with the diagnosis. In Western culture, we place a value of being independent and autonomous entirely, and you may try to behave according to the norms of our culture. This partly explains why you tried to conceal any signs that you may not be coping, have changed from how you were before, or you may need support from others. In this attempt to conceal

Parkinson's from others, you may have started avoiding going out or contributing to conversations. But where does all this lead to?

By avoiding being with others, you are missing out opportunities to explore your thoughts and see them through another's lenses. By repeatedly avoiding social engagements and proactively seeking others' company, you are shrinking your network. We humans are social animals, and we are happier when we are with others. Social isolation and loneliness leads to poorer health and well-being.

We all have our 'go-to' ways to deal with anxious feelings. Maybe you try to suppress unpleasant feelings with distraction, watching TV, sleeping, or playing video games. And it does work, at least in the short term. The problem is that with these techniques you do not add anything into your life. You subtract, you survive, there is comfort but do these activities and way of living propel you live your life to the full?

There are other ways that you could try. Not every day, not all the time but if your 'go-to' strategies are all about the distractions it might be good occasionally to try something different to see if that would work for you. Mindfulness could provide some alterative coping strategies you could keep in your back pocket (see a quick mindfulness exercise in the next section of this chapter). Mindfulness slows down the breathing and focuses the brain to the now. This helps with the physical manifestation of anxiety, so physically you are calmer and cognitively you have better clarity of what is needed to do and focus your attention. You can see similar positive effects with self-care practices, like exercise and massages; these can alleviate symptoms and also enhance well-being.

Social connections can also be valuable, especially if you're feeling that anxiety or Parkinson's affects your social identity. Indeed, studies of those with long-term health conditions show social networks can benefit well-being even if made up of 'weak' ties outside of family and friends, for example, by joining an exercise group, dance course, choir, or Parkinson's group. However, some people may feel reluctant joining a formal support group with other people who might have more severe Parkinson's symptoms than themselves, which they might feel would heighten anxiety about disease progression.

Cognitive behavioural therapy is a form of psychological treatment that helps people understand their thoughts and behaviours. It is based in the idea that our thoughts, feelings, and actions are connected, so negative thinking patterns can lead to distress and harmful behaviour. In 2021, the British Psychological Society published a monograph on psychological interventions for people with neurological conditions including, Parkinson's and concluded that cognitive behavioural therapy has the most consistent positive effect, and it has positive effects on depression when delivered individually, in groups, over the phone, or online. However, adherence to computer-based programmes has been a challenge. Pychoeducation programmes might also help people adjust after deep brain stimulation.

Not everyone will align or find cognitive behavioural therapy helpful, as its main aim is to challenge thoughts and thought pattern. Some people with Parkinson's might find that these approaches do not always take into account that the anxiety is part of the condition and not only a response.

Alternative therapies are also becoming more popular, approaches that do not challenge thoughts or feelings, but accept them as valid manifestations of how things are now. It is what we call third-wave behavioural therapies, such as acceptance and commitment therapy. This approach builds on second-wave cognitive behavioural therapy but instead of testing and changing thoughts, the therapy focuses on supporting psychological flexibility and identifying ways to live in accordance with one's values, despite adversity.

Due to the progressive nature of the disease, people with Parkinson's as well as carers continually reframe their acceptance over time (Tuijt et al., 2020). Although this is described as a gradual process involving denial, sadness, and anger, trying to have a positive mindset and outlook on life was recognised as an important way of trying to live as well as possible. Accepting the disease as well as accepting the possible future that awaits people with Parkinson's and their carers can bring about stress and anxiety. In order to stop worrying about the future, acceptance can direct the focus on day-to-day life and valuing what you could do and found enjoyable (Tuijt et al., 2020). Acceptance, as a term, might have negative connotations for some, but what it means is that you are open to feelings, experiences, and symptoms, you let them be as they are. If we stop the struggle of suppressing or altering experiences, feelings and symptoms, we have a better view of what we are dealing with, which then gives us more control over how we would like to respond to these situations, feelings and symptoms. Maybe you let things be while you direct your attention at something that is more important to you, maybe you discuss issues with a loved one and come up with a plan of action, of what needs to be done and who can help with things, maybe you decide not to do anything about uncomfortable thoughts. Whatever the decision, it is a conscious choice rather than a reaction. Accepting by being open is a simple concept but difficult to do, it needs time, and it might feel it is not always possible.

2.3 HOW TO STAY AWARE OF EMOTIONS, THOUGHTS, AND OTHER EXPERIENCES?

Being present in our lives will help us get more out of it and make living fulfilling and meaningful, rather than sleepwalking through life, feeling constantly distracted, living in the past or in the future, get ourselves busy for the sake of being busy. But then life is passing by and we are not really in it and we are not in control of how we spent it but rather reacting to whatever the environment is throwing at us. We've all been there. And sometimes, it is OK, we are in a season of life that we can't avoid it. We can't be present all the time but the aim here is to 'wake up', more frequently, to stay in the 'present' mode a little bit longer.

Mindfulness is a word we used when we want to describe being present and aware, but it is a little more complex than that. Jon Kabat-Zinn defined mindfulness as:

Paying attention . . . on purpose, in the present moment, and non-judgementally.

The definition highlights two key ingredients of mindfulness: a cognitive aspect – paying attention, staying focused, and doing so intentionally – and a relational aspect – meeting experiences with kindness, patience, and without judgement. Mindfulness, in this sense, is a skill, a way of relating to yourself, your body, and the world that can be cultivated over time. For people living with Parkinson's, this can offer a powerful tool to navigate the emotional and physical ups and downs of the condition.

Everyone has the capacity to be mindful, even if it does not come easily at first. While some people may be naturally good at focusing their attention, they might find it harder to be gentle or non-judgemental with themselves. Others might be very compassionate, but find their attention drifts or scatters easily, especially when under stress or living with symptoms like fatigue or anxiety. Mindfulness brings together attention and attitude. It is about what we are focusing on, and *how* we relate to what we find. It is not about achieving a blank mind or pushing away thoughts and feelings. Rather, it is about noticing what is happening in the moment and choosing how to respond, with awareness and kindness.

Mindfulness training usually begins with learning to anchor attention to the present moment using something simple and bodily, like the breath, the sensation of the feet on the floor, or the sounds around you. These anchors are always available, and they help pull us back from spiralling into the past or future. This can offer a brief sense of steadiness, but it is not always easy, especially when there's physical pain, tremor, or emotional distress. That is why practice, patience, and self-compassion are central to mindfulness.

Let's try a short practice that helps anchor your attention to the breath.

MINDFUL BREATHING

Find a position that you can sustain comfortably the next 5 minutes. Shift your attention so that you are aware of your feet on the floor, feel your body in contact with the chair or the surface you are on, holding and supporting you, you are rising up from this surface to an alert and comfortable position.

Now become aware of the fact that you are breathing. Don't try to breathe in a particular way, just notice how you breathe naturally. Simply feel the sensations of the breath as it moves through your body. How does the air feel as it comes in through your nose? Does it get warmer as you breathe out? What parts of your body move with your breath? Can you feel sensations in your abdomen, chest, neck, throat, or nose?

If at any point, you notice that your mind has wandered away from the breath, into thinking, or distracted by a sound, or perhaps drawn to a sensation in the body, remember that this is not a problem – it is what minds do and as soon as you realise that you have wandered away, gently come back to the anchor of the breath, notice its rhythm, if there are any pauses between your breath. Focus on the sensations of the waves of the breath, breathing in and breathing out, your breath coming in, and going out.

Take a moment to notice how you feel after doing this activity. If you ever feel like your mind is getting caught up in worries or negative thoughts, you can always return to activities like this to bring your mind back to the present moment.

Over the past few decades, mindfulness-based approaches have become increasingly common in physical and mental healthcare. A key catalyst for this growth was the development of mindfulness-based stress reduction, an eight-week group programme introduced in the 1980s in the U.S. healthcare system. Designed by Jon Kabat-Zinn, mindfulness-based stress reduction was initially created to support people living with chronic physical conditions worsened by stress, such as chronic pain, eczema, and irritable bowel syndrome. Its standardised structure made it well suited for research, which led to a growing evidence base supporting its use across diverse healthcare settings.

Building on the mindfulness-based stress reduction model, researchers at the Oxford Mindfulness Centre developed mindfulness-based cognitive therapy, which integrates mindfulness practice with cognitive therapy techniques. Mindfulness-based cognitive therapy was originally developed to help people with recurrent depression, aiming to prevent relapse by helping individuals recognise and disengage from habitual patterns of negative thinking (Kuyken et al., 2016). Typically, this course includes around 80% mindfulness training and 20% cognitive elements.

Even though the two mindfulness programmes have some differences, the mindfulness-based stress reduction focuses more on stress responses, whereas the mindfulness-based cognitive therapy focuses on unhelpful thoughts. They are very similar and when synthesising evidence from the literature, we usually combine the different versions of the mindfulness courses. Vidyamala Burch has also created a mindfulness programme specifically for those experiencing long-term physical conditions, called Breathworks. You can find out more about the approach and lot of free resources on the Breathworks website.

These 8-week courses consist of 2-hour-long weekly meetings and daily mindfulness meditation practice (about 45 minutes a day). The mindfulness courses focus on finding a new way to relate to thoughts and experiences and to accept them as passing events that do not necessarily represent a state of reality. The mechanism at its core is not about eliminating pain or stress, but about changing our relationship to them. By cultivating awareness, kindness, and acceptance, we can respond to discomfort in a more adaptive way, reducing the secondary suffering that often comes from resistance or reactivity.

Living with Parkinson's can be challenging, not only because of the physical symptoms but also because of how we *react* to those symptoms. Our thoughts, emotional responses, and actions can sometimes add another layer of distress, often without us even realising it. Mindfulness invites us to bring gentle, non-judging awareness to whatever we're experiencing, right here, right now. By learning to meet our sensations, thoughts, and feelings with openness rather than resistance, we begin to shift how we relate to them. This doesn't mean ignoring the hard stuff or pretending everything's fine. Instead, we are learning to be with our experience in a way that's more spacious and less reactive.

Many reactions to symptoms, like tension, fear, frustration, or self-criticism, happen so quickly and automatically that they become fused with the symptoms themselves. For example, a sudden tremor might instantly trigger a thought like 'This is getting worse', followed by a wave of anxiety. The anxiety may tighten the body, which then makes the tremor feel even more distressing. This is how a fusion can form.

Through mindfulness, we can notice these patterns more clearly. We might start to see the difference between the physical sensation (the symptom) and our mental and emotional reactions to it. With practice, this opens the door to responding more skilfully, noticing what's happening, pausing, and choosing a response rather than being swept away. While it is natural to pay attention to symptoms, constantly scanning the body or mind can amplify distress and keep us stuck in a loop of worry or discomfort.

Mindfulness helps us shift our focus intentionally and experience thoughts as just thoughts and sensations as just sensations without immediately assuming the worst. This subtle shift can weaken the cycle of negative interpretation and over-attention that often comes with chronic health conditions. In essence, mindfulness does not aim to eliminate symptoms, but it can reduce the suffering that surrounds them. By learning to relate differently to the ups and downs of our condition, we may find a little more space, ease, and steadiness within the experience of living with Parkinson's.

Mindfulness-based approaches cultivate acceptance of the situation as it is right now, balancing those aspects of it which cannot be changed with mindful action towards values, where such change is possible. This can be immensely helpful in supporting skilful self-management. In many conditions, symptoms vary from day to day and moment to moment. Being aware of these changes can help us to respond flexibly to them, including doing nothing (e.g. not taking extra rest) when that is the most skilful thing to do. Learning how to be kinder towards ourselves can reduce the frustration and self-criticism which often accompanies adjustment to physical changes and limitations.

Mindfulness courses can help reduce distress but especially depression. In a study published in PLOS Medicine, Galante and colleagues gathered data from 136 mindfulness trials that included 11,605 participants. When compared with no intervention, people in the mindfulness groups showed improved depression, with no statistically significant evidence on improving anxiety, distress, and well-being (Galante et al., 2021). Moreover, when the comparison of the mindfulness groups was with non–active controls, the participants of the mindfulness groups showed improved depressive symptoms but no other outcomes. The National Institute for Health and Care Excellence (NICE) guidance supports the use of mindfulness to prevent relapses for people diagnosed with chronic depression. In terms of long–term conditions, we have evidence for significant improvements in psychological well-being across different conditions. However, the evidence is inconclusive when it comes to improvements in physical health measures, except pain. Even though we do have some evidence on mindfulness helping improve pain, the evidence is not robust enough, and NICE guidelines (2021) for chronic pain do not recommend mindfulness as a primary psychological treatment, however, they acknowledge its potential and identify it as an important area for further research.

It is important to underline that mindfulness is not a psychological therapy in the traditional sense; it helps people to stay present. However, it does not have other active techniques used in traditional therapies. Also, contrary to popular beliefs, mindfulness is not about positive thinking and is not a relaxation technique. Mindfulness teaches people to stay present, observe emotions, thoughts, and symptoms as they are without judging them and without wanting them to be different. Mindfulness talks about not being too attached to anything that is positive or negative because everything is transient, everything comes and goes, and if we are attached to something that is positive when it goes, we will suffer, so instead we hold our experiences lightly. Also, when people expecting to find mindfulness relaxing have a rude awakening when they first practice.

Trying to keep your mind constantly in the present by focusing, for example, on your breath or a part of your body is effortful and can be uncomfortable. Eventually, some people find the mindfulness practices relaxing, which is a nice side effect, but this is not always true.

With Parkinson's, there can be a number of things on your mind, and the below activity is a simple way to shift your focus from the problem that's bothering you and to connect with the present moment. Doing this can give you a break and help you feel more grounded. The three-minute breathing space activity has three steps, and you can spend around a minute on each step. It is easy enough to practice whenever you need to or regularly through your day, for example, while you are waiting for a kettle to boil or the microwave to warm up your lunch. In the mindfulness groups, I have run with people with multiple sclerosis and Parkinson's, this activity is by far the most popular. By practicing mindfulness activities like the below you are strengthening the muscles of attention and compassion and eventually the effects will spill outside of practice, initially for a few minutes after practicing the activity and then more and more, until you get large chunks of your day that you feel centred and kind towards yourself and others.

And here is how you do it. You start by finding a comfortable posture, perhaps closing your eyes if that's comfortable for you.

The 3-minute breathing space

Step 1: seeing what's going on in your mind and body right now. What thoughts are around? What feelings are there? Not trying to change anything, but being aware of what is already there. Notice any sensations in the body? Notice your feet on the ground, or, if you're sitting or lying down, notice the surface you are on; your clothes against your body and the air against your skin.

Step 2: bringing your attention to the breath. Focus on sensations of the breath on the abdomen. Tuning in to the physical sensations of the in-breath for its full duration and the out-breath for its full duration. Notice the cool air flowing in through your nose as you inhale and the warm air as you exhale, as you breathe in and out. If your mind wanders, simply acknowledge where it went and gently escort it back to the breath.

Step 3: expand the focus of your awareness around the breath to the whole body, as if the whole body was breathing now. Become aware of the whole length of your body, your face, sensations on the surface of your skin and sensations inside your body. Holding in your awareness all the sensations in your body right now, just as they are at this moment. Gently broaden your awareness to notice your whole experience and the space around you.

And finally, you gently open your eyes.

Think of this activity as an hourglass shape. The first step, your awareness is wide on what is happening at that moment for you, the second step narrows down to the breath and focuses the mind and the third step your awareness expands once again to take in all your surroundings. Before you open your eyes, you can also set an intention, what do you want to do next or how you want to show up to what you are about to do.

It is likely in the previous activity you found your mind wandering. Expect the mind to wander. The mind naturally drifts, this is completely normal. Often, it wanders to the past (regret, rumination), or into the future (worry, planning). For you, mind-wandering may include anxious thoughts about progression, health appointments, or the emotional weight of what is been lost or may change.

This wandering is not a problem in itself. In fact, recognising that your attention has drifted is a moment of mindfulness, something to acknowledge with kindness. No need to fight the thoughts or analyse them, just notice, let go, and come back. This skill, of noticing and returning, can be developed through short, repeated practice. Over time, it can help reduce emotional reactivity, increase focus, and make room for more flexibility in how we respond to challenges.

Mindfulness teaches us to stay aware of emotions, thoughts, and other experiences, approach our experiences with acceptance, not in a passive way, but with openness and curiosity. When we reduce judgement, even painful moments become more manageable. As the Buddhists put it, 'Pain is hard enough. But pain + resistance = suffering.' Mindfulness does not aim to eliminate difficulty, but it can ease the additional suffering that comes from fighting or fearing what we feel. It helps us remember that emotions, just like thoughts, are temporary and can be witnessed with care. Mindfulness doesn't require you to get rid of difficult thoughts or feelings, it invites you to relate to them differently. This approach may be especially valuable for people with Parkinson's, where physical symptoms and emotional challenges often do not have quick fixes. Mindfulness helps us relate to ourselves with more kindness, patience, and resilience.

2.4 HOW TO STAY OPEN TO EMOTIONS, FEELINGS, AND OTHER EXPERIENCES?

One key part of acceptance and commitment therapy (Hayes, 2004) is called openness or acceptance. In this chapter, we will discuss the concept as well as some activities originated by Hayes, the founder of acceptance and commitment therapy, but adapted to be more relevant in the context of Parkinson's. Being open means being willing to experience events, thoughts, and feelings as they are, without trying to suppress or avoid them. When we are open, we might also experience uncomfortable, frustrating, or painful experiences. Being open does not mean we have to try to like the experience or see the positive side of those experiences. We are simply acknowledging that they exist.

Being open means dropping your resistance or struggle with unpleasant thoughts and feelings. We can allow them to be there, we don't have to like these thoughts and feelings. They will likely come and go, but by letting them be there and being open, we can free up the energy we were using to fight them, to start doing what matters to us. This is what it means to be open or practice openness.

We all experience worries and sadness from time to time; they are a normal part of life, but sometimes these thoughts and feelings become too much for us, and we might have trouble focusing on other things. We might find that we spend our time worrying rather than getting on with things that matter to us.

The below brief breathing exercise could help you to 'let go' or 'unhook' from these negative thoughts so that you feel calmer and can start to focus on other, more enjoyable things and feel more in control of your life. Read through the instructions once. Then close your eyes if that feels OK and try to practice the exercise.

Breathing exercise

For the next 5 minutes, find a comfortable place to sit. The first step to doing this is to begin to notice our thoughts, which is not something we often do, so try following these instructions and see what you notice. Close your eyes, if that is comfortable, or turn your gaze toward the floor before you and focus on your breathing. Take a few deep breaths in and out, using this opportunity to release any areas of tension from the body; release any tightness, perhaps the muscles in the face, the jaw, neck, or shoulders. Use each exhale to let go of any stress or tension.

Focus on your breathing as best you can, even if just for a few breaths. You will soon notice that thoughts are popping into your head, even if you are trying to focus on your breathing. When you notice a thought arise, label it as a thought. For example, each time you notice a thought, just silently, inwardly note to yourself, 'that's a thought'. If you would like, you can be more specific. For example, if you notice a judgmental thought arise such as 'I'm not good at this' or 'This is boring', label it 'that's a judgement' or if you notice a thought such as 'I must remember to buy some milk', you can label it 'that is planning'. If you notice a thought from the past, you might label it 'remembering' or 'predicting' and so on.

If your mind gets repeatedly drawn into the story created by your thoughts or if any thoughts are difficult to let go, remember that you can always come back to your breath to anchor your awareness to the present moment before returning, if you choose, to observing your thoughts.

Continue to notice the thoughts that come into your head. Notice what thoughts are difficult to let go of; these thoughts are likely ones you are attached to or hooked on. When we do not attach much to a thought, it tends to be easier to release.

Labelling or observing our thoughts is one way to stop becoming too concerned with these thoughts. It can help us understand that these are not facts but merely thoughts, and we can then try to take a step back and let go of them. Some people find it helpful when doing this exercise to think of their thoughts as leaves in a stream. When sitting for a few minutes to practice being open to your experience, you could instead imagine this scene. See yourself sitting by the side of a stream on a warm, sunny day. You see leaves floating by on the water, and then you put each of your thoughts into a sentence that will be written on a leaf. If you would rather see your thoughts as images, that is ok too. Try to watch the leaves floating along with one thought after another without interruption.

The tricky part is that you will find this difficult to do at first. When you realise, as you certainly will, that the stream has disappeared and that you have become lost in your thoughts, back up a few moments and connect with what you were doing at the point that the stream disappeared. When you get back to where you were, simply restart the process, putting your thoughts on hold until the next time you get lost, and so on. If at some stage you begin thinking 'I'm not getting this right' or 'This is too difficult', then just put those types of thoughts on a leaf and send them down the stream as well.

This breathing exercise, where you sit, observe and label your thoughts, or imagine your thoughts floating down a river, not only helps to become more aware of your thoughts and feelings, but you will hold more control over them, so they will not interfere with your plans and with who you want to be. You are like a bus driver, and you want to go somewhere. Your thoughts and feelings are the passengers who have their own ideas of where they want to go. They do not always want to go where you want to go, and when you do not go their way, they let you know about it. They may confront, hassle, or threaten you. They essentially bully you, so you do what they say. You choose not to go where <u>you</u> want to go, and they settle down, into the back of the bus and out of sight. In the meantime, you're driving around in circles and not going anywhere in particular, just driving aimlessly. But the only power they have over you is the power you give them. You are the driver, yet you trade your control over the bus to keep the passengers away.

Maybe you are experiencing a situation like this. You may also have scary, intimidating passengers – these are thoughts, feelings, sensations, pain, urges, memories, and the like. They go where you go, or stay where you stay. Can you see the sense in which these thoughts and feelings can take over where you want to go? Thoughts like 'Exercise is for fit people', 'I'm too slow, people in the shops will be annoyed with me', 'Parkinson's doesn't let me enjoy my hobbies'.

If you make an active choice to go where you want to go, you may still hear the passengers in the background, but their voices will gradually get softer. Their voices may keep popping up again, and you hear them, but make the choice to go in the direction you want to go. The passengers can scream. They can yell. They can do whatever they want. They might get on the bus when they want and get off of the bus when they want. That is totally up to them. But you control the bus, and you get to drive it where you want to go.

Openness is the willingness to experience thoughts and emotions as they are, without trying to avoid or control them. Being open doesn't mean liking difficult experiences; it means acknowledging them without resistance. When we don't spend time and energy to 'fight' experiences, feelings and thoughts, we have more time and energy to devote to what truly matters in life. When you catch yourself getting hooked in an experience, thought, or feeling and you replay it again and again, in your mind's eye, acknowledge it, maybe label it and letting them pass like leaves floating down a stream. Even something as simple as labelling a feeling ('This is sadness' or 'This is frustration') can shift the relationship to it. This small moment of mindfulness creates choice, allowing us to respond with more self-kindness and less automatic reactivity. Practising this technique regularly, especially during moments of overwhelm, can help you regain clarity and stay anchored in the present. In short, openness means allowing uncomfortable thoughts and feelings to exist, without letting them dictate your actions, so you can live more fully in line with your values.

Some types of thinking support us, like planning or reflecting. But when thoughts become repetitive or emotionally charged (e.g. self-criticism, catastrophic predictions), they can deepen distress. This is especially relevant for people with Parkinson's who may experience mood fluctuations or feelings of hopelessness. Mindfulness training helps build awareness of these mental habits, so we can learn to shift attention *before* they spiral. We learn when to lean into emotional experience (with support), and when it is healthier to rest attention in the body or the senses.

While mindfulness begins with physical anchors like breathing or movement, over time it also brings greater awareness to mental activity, thoughts, images, emotions, and memories. This is where deeper healing often begins. We become more familiar with the patterns of the mind, the stories we tell to ourselves about ourselves, and learn not to automatically follow every thought.

All of us have self-evaluations, stories of who we are. Some of our stories are positive and some are negative. Stories that reflect sentiments like 'I am worthless' or 'I am a failure' can stop us from taking care of ourselves or seeking what we want out of life. Positive sounding sentiments like 'I am independent', 'I can look after myself', or 'I am successful, or wise', can stop us from seeking support when we need it, or from recognising, taking responsibility, and learning from mistakes. The trouble with self-evaluations or stories, whether they are positive or negative, is that they can often block us from doing what we want to do, if we over-identify or take them too seriously. Even 'a Parkinson's patient' can be a kind of self-imposed restriction, if you see it as the essence of who you are.

Let's now look at an activity that brings a wider focus away from those stories. You can first read the instructions of this activity and then practice it with eyes closed or with a soft focus on a particular spot or you can ask someone to read this for you while you are practicing.

Stories about me

First, notice your breath. Notice the sensations of your breath as it moves in and out of your body. Notice that there is the breath and there is you noticing it. There is a distinction between the breath and the 'you' who notices the breath. Your breath constantly changes, sometimes it is shallow, sometimes deep, sometimes quick and sometimes slow. Yet you, who notices does not change.

You are separate from the experiences you are having. This is what we mean by your observing self. Now, notice your thoughts, notice as they come and go. Notice that you are noticing your thoughts. Your thoughts may change, but you, who observes the thoughts does not change. When you were younger you had thoughts that are different from the ones you have today. We learn new things and sometimes we find that thoughts we used to believe are not true. Notice that your thoughts change over time, but it is always the same you.

Your mind is unlikely to agree with what is being said here or will try to analyse it. When you notice your mind doing this, simply notice that you are noticing it at the same time.

Now, notice your body and any sensations you feel. Then notice that you are noticing sensations of your body. The body is always changing. Sometimes you feel well and sometimes you feel poorly, sometimes there are aches and pains in one part and sometimes they are in another part or sometimes these do not register at all. Yet you, who notices these sensations or the absence of sensations, does not change.

Notice if there is any particular emotion or mood present for you right now. It could be curiosity, calmness, boredom, anticipation, or the like. Then notice that you are noticing these feelings. There is a distinction or separation between the emotional feelings that you can detect and you who can detect them. If there is anything we can say about moods and emotions, it is that they are ever changing. Sometimes we are happy and sometimes we are sad. A feeling of anxiety or anger may come, and it will always pass eventually. During all of these occasions is the same, unchanging, you.

Now let's focus on the roles we have. There are roles that you are taking on at this very moment. You can take on the role of a reader of a psychology book, at other times you are in the role of mother, father, brother, sister, son or daughter, friend, competitor, customer, worker, and so on. Then notice that you are noticing your roles. Our roles are always changing, and they might have changed since being diagnosed with Parkinson's, but the person – you are still the same.

What does all this mean? Although you have thoughts, sensations, feelings, and roles, you are not just your thoughts, sensations, feelings, and roles. They are always changing and you, who observes them is steady. You are not defined by your thoughts, feelings, and roles but are separate from your thoughts and feelings, bigger, like a container of your thoughts, feelings, and roles.

Take a few moments after you complete this activity to notice some of the reactions, thoughts, feelings, or questions you have from doing this activity. Some people find this activity very moving, others may not. The key is not to over-analyse what your mind says about doing this activity, but focus on your experience of being separate and bigger than your thoughts, sensations, and feelings. Over time, this practice helps loosen the grip of self-criticism, worry, or fear, without denying the reality of the experience. Another, metaphor we usually use in acceptance and commitment therapy is picturing yourself as a mountain, and your feelings, thoughts, and physical symptoms as the weather around the mountain. You are a solid unchanged presence but the weather around you might change; seasons come and go but you remain calm and centred.

2.5 HOW TO STAY ENGAGED WITH YOUR MEANINGFUL ACTIVITIES AND TASKS?

Finding space in your day-to-day life to engage with meaningful activities can be difficult. Acceptance and commitment therapy (Hayes, 2004) places a lot of focus on identifying values and aligning daily activities with values. Here, we will discuss the concepts of values and some activities originated by Hayes (2004), but adapted to be relevant in the context of Parkinson's. Perhaps, you already know what is meaningful and brings most fulfilment and what drains your energy and does not add much value in your life. The question is how you prioritise those activities that rarely feel as urgent over the many other things you need to do to manage Parkinson's along with keeping everything in your life organised and working. We all had the feeling of a huge list of things we would like to do; we prioritise the most urgent that have to do with health and also involves others and then there is not much time or energy left for the things that will make life feel full and meaningful.

Let's spend some time thinking about values. Imagine you are 10 years older than you currently are, and you are celebrating your birthday (or you are celebrating a milestone birthday in the future). Let's first set the scene. What do you see around you, what does it sound like, smell like, and feel like? On this notable day, you have a moment for reflection on the past. Is there something in your life you spent too much time worrying about? Is there something you spent too little time doing? If you could go back in time to the person you are today, is there something you would do differently? This could be things like 'I wish I spent more time with family' or 'I would try and learn more new skills and hobbies'. From these reflections, you can recognise what your values are, things like family or relationships, desire to learn or challenge yourself. Take a moment to think about what your values might be.

A value is a direction in life that you would like to follow for example, being a loving partner or a helpful colleague. Values are important because following them helps you make choices and guides you towards what you want.

Now, let's go through different areas in your life. Try to think of your values in relation to each of these areas. If you don't have any values for a particular area that's okay, everyone's situation is different. Remember there are no 'correct' values, they are simply things that are important to you and give your life direction and meaning.

1. **Relationships.** Try to think about your close relationships and also your relationships in general with people you meet. What is important to you? Is it things like nurturing your relationships? Or perhaps being honest with yourself or others or kind or loving? Your value could be connection: to be fully present with others or to be friendly, companionable, or agreeable towards others.
2. **Health and well-being.** This may be difficult to think about because of having Parkinson's, but it is still important to do.

Focus on what is important to you in terms of your health. Perhaps it is about trying to manage your Parkinson's symptoms as best as you can. Or doing some kind of physical activity, whatever your level of ability is. Broaden this area of your life to also think about your mental health. This may already be a value for you because you have decided to read this book. Your value could be self-care: to look after your health and well-being and get your needs met or mindfulness: to be conscious of, open to and curious about your here and now experience.

3. **Work and leisure.** This may include things like your job, your voluntary work, or even looking after the house. Leisure activities can be anything you do for fun or pleasure. What do you value in this area of your life? Maybe it is things like providing for your family or making a contribution to society in some way however small. It could be learning new things or being able to see the fun side of life. For example, your value could be industrious: to be industrious, hard-working, and dedicated, or fun: to seek, create, and engage in fun-filled activities.

Before you carry on reading, take a few moments to reflect on the above questions. Did you notice any new values that came up this time? Or did this activity help you fine tune a value you had already identified? Perhaps, make a mental, written, or recorded note of your values in relation to each of these areas of your life. Don't worry if you can't think of any values right now or if your values change over time. You can earmark this page and come back to it later. You might have a large list of values, but let's focus on your top three or five values.

But why values are so important? Let me give you an example. Think of something you've done that was so difficult, you hoped you'd never have to do it again. Now consider if you would do it again if the health of someone close to you depended on it – your children's, or your parents', or your best friend's. What if I said that for every time you do this again, your kid, parent, or best friend can live a year without suffering any health problems. What would you say? Think about this and keep the answer to yourself.

If you found that having more to gain made the difficult thing more possible to do, this is like what values do – they make our choices worth it. There are many things that we do that carry costs, particularly with Parkinson's in the picture. For example, if you want to go somewhere or do a particular activity, you may need to ask someone for help or use a piece of equipment to help you. The time or effort or preparation or potential frustration in doing some of these activities is very real and can stop you from doing them in the first place. This is where our values come in, the things we choose to do and the costs they carry are ultimately for us to decide. If we are clear on what we might have to gain, we can be more certain about doing the action.

Sometimes we do things that are moving us **away** from our values. Moving away from the life outcome you want, acting ineffectively, behaving unlike the person you want to be. And then, there are other activities that are moving us **towards** what we value. Moving towards the life outcome you want, acting effectively, and behaving like the person you want to be. Notice that this moving towards what is important often includes moving towards things that are difficult, and there is often no getting around that. The power in values is that they clarify what's at stake and what's to gain. They orient us and change running away from difficulties into moving towards what's important.

Values are choices we make about the kind of person we want to be and the kind of life we want to lead. Once we know what they are, we can create goals to help us live in a more meaningful way. Both values and goals are important and related, but there is a slight difference. Values can be ongoing, like being a loving partner, or maintaining physical fitness. Goals are achievements we can succeed in, like getting married, celebrating a 20th anniversary, joining a gym or class, or getting outside for some fresh air for 20 minutes three times this week. Values are like a compass pointing us in the direction we want to go, while goals are like a signpost on the journey towards this direction.

Why do we need to pay attention to our values and goals? Values and goals can be very useful as they give us direction and help us focus on what is meaningful. This can feel positive and energise us even in difficult situations. But how can values help us? How do we align with them? Sometimes thinking about our values and planning the relevant actions can feel quite big, unclear, or too difficult. This can stop us from getting started in the first place. Let's work through this step by step.

Goals are more likely to lead to success if they have the following qualities referred to as **SMART** which stands for: **S**pecific, **M**easurable, **A**chievable, **R**elevant, **T**ime-framed.

Let's go through each of these points with examples.

Specific: Goals should be precise and action-oriented so that you know just what you need to do and under what circumstances. 'Get fit' is a vague goal, while 'walk 500 meters at least three times per week' is specific.

Measurable: 'Measurable' is another way to say that there needs to be a way that you can identify when your goal has been reached. If your goal is to exercise at least four times per week, for 15 minutes each time, for example, you can place a calendar on your refrigerator, make a check mark each time you exercise, and count how many times you have done that at the end of the week.

Achievable: If goals are set too high, they can feel impossible or discouraging, or can set you up for failure. At the same time, goals set too low can feel as if they are not meaningful. It is useful to consider whether you have the skills you need, time, money, and opportunity to reach your goals. What is achievable will be different for everyone.

Relevant: It is useful to identify what it is about your particular goals that make them desirable and important to you. We have already done some work to identify our values earlier in this chapter, so goals that are linked to your values are already relevant to you.

Time-framed: It will help to set a deadline for each goal you set. We all need deadlines at times to assure that we do not put off doing the things we want to do. Setting a deadline gives you a clear target to meet and makes your goal 'time-specific'.

Try to use the SMART tool to set a new goal for yourself. Make sure it is specific, measurable, attainable, relevant, and time-framed.

Setting up a SMART goal

Use the space below to record your new goal. Think about how you might complete the following statements:

1. (Specific) The specific goal I want to achieve is _____
2. (Measurable) I will know my goal has been reached when _____
3. (Achievable) To make my goal attainable I will need _____ (resources or skills)
4. (Relevant) This goal is important to me because _____
5. (Time-framed) I will achieve my goal by this date _____

Another way to ensure the goals will be achieved is by setting small steps towards those goals. Sometimes thinking about our values and planning the relevant actions can feel quite big, unclear or too difficult. This can stop us from getting started in the first place. Let's work through this step by step.

First, think about one of your values that you would like to work on right now. I am not asking you to make a commitment or goal right now nor to plan an action, just to think about the long-term picture. Try to identify a commitment or goal you could make in line with your value, possibly to put into action within the next year or so. For example, if your value is to get connected with nature, your goal for the year could be to create a wildlife friendly corner in the garden and be able to observe and enjoy the wildlife that use this space.

Then, from there, try to identify a commitment or goal that is consistent with your value, and maybe something small and simple which you could do within the next month or so. With the same example, your goal might be to buy certain plants or to create a pond in your garden.

Now try to identify a commitment or goal that you put into action to move towards your value in the next week or so. This could be for example, buying some seeds or making a decision about how you want to design your garden space.

Lastly, try to identify a commitment or goal you could begin in line with your value in the next day or so. This could be something small like reading up or watching a television programme about gardening.

Now try to do this with your own value that you selected. Identify a commitment that you could put into action in a year, then in the next month, next week, and the next day. Notice your thoughts and feelings as you consider this commitment. What does your mind say? What shows up in your feelings? You may notice potential barriers that automatically show up the moment we want to aim for something we care about, both big and small, far ahead and near in time. Would you be willing to set a goal and take your small step, follow through with your smallest commitment, today or tomorrow?

When it comes to setting goals, we often focus on the positive aspects of reaching them and how achieving them makes us feel good. But our chances of success will be higher if we are also aware of the potential barriers or things that might interfere with our plans.

Take a moment to focus on a goal you have set for yourself and what could get in the way of achieving it. These barriers might be practical such as not having enough time or money, or symptom-related where Parkinson's symptoms make something difficult to do.

As you identify each barrier, try to think how you might be able to overcome it or consider how you might incorporate this barrier into your plan for achieving your goal. For example, if you're trying to be more physically active but finding time to do it or even remembering to do it is tricky, then your strategy could be setting a reminder or asking someone to remind you or planning a specific time for it to help you get into the routine of doing the physical activity. If a Parkinson's-related symptom is a barrier to achieving your goal, then your strategy could be modifying the activity, asking for help, or even pacing yourself and giving yourself more time to reach your goal. For example, if fatigue gets in the way later in the day, you may want to break down your goal and schedule it in small chunks earlier in the day.

If achieving your goal involves both pleasant and potentially unpleasant experiences, you might plan to use your 'openness' or 'present-moment awareness' skills to overcome these barriers, as we saw in the previous sections. For example, if your goal is to meet your friend at a café but the barrier is being self-conscious of your symptoms in public places, one strategy could be practicing openness to acknowledge and work through these thoughts and feelings. You can practice distancing or unhooking from these unhelpful thoughts by labelling them. If these feelings are too overwhelming, you can start with small steps like meeting at a quieter place or at a less busy time of day.

These different suggestions are to help you think about potential barriers and to acknowledge and plan for them as you think about setting your goals. Achieving your goals can take some effort, but it is important to remember why you are doing them. Each time you encounter a potential barrier and persist, you're engaged in what we call committed action. You're moving closer to your values and to the life you want to live.

Each goal is a little step which will help you move towards what you want from life. You also need to be aware of any difficult thoughts and feelings that get in your way, such as anxiety, fear of failure, and all those thoughts about it being too hard or why it won't work. But you also need to make sure you live the best possible life today, even while these goals are not yet achieved. Because you don't know how long it will take you to achieve these goals. It could take a long time and there are no guarantees. So, you can also focus on ways you can improve your life on a day-to-day basis; to live the richest fullest life possible here and now even though some of these goals may be a long way off.

Now you understand the importance of values, have identified your values, and set some goals that align with these values and identify how to overcome any barriers in your way. Here are some tips to help keep you motivated and on track with your progress in the coming days. You can remember this using the acronym VISA.

V stands for **V**alue actions. This means two things – first, literally remember that action is how results are achieved, there is power in action, and second, motivate actions by using values as your guide. **I** stands for **I**dentify and plan for challenges. For example, you could regularly practice some of the mindfulness activities earlier in this chapter. The letter **S** stands for **S**eek support for your goals. Tell someone you care about what is important to you and what your goals are. See if you can involve this person when you're working on your goals. And the last letter **A** stands for **A**pply reminders. Schedule your goals into your diary or put an alarm on your phone. Place a statement about your values or goals somewhere you will see it every day.

Checking-in activity

After you have identified your values and perhaps set up some goals, you can periodically spend a few minutes reflecting on whether your activities align with your values, by answering the prompts below, you can do this mentally or record your answers in a notebook or record them in your phone as voice memos to come back to.

Sit in a comfortable position and start to think about everything you did yesterday. Spend some time reviewing your activities, almost as if a documentary was being made about your life and what you did yesterday.

Now think about the values you identified earlier. Which of yesterday's activities took you away from behaving like the kind of person you want to be? And which of yesterday's activities moved you towards the life outcome you want, behaving like the person you want to be? For example, if your value is to keep learning new things and growing, turning down an opportunity to do something because it was out of your comfort zone took you away from this value. Alternatively, trying that task even though it made you feel a little uncomfortable, took you closer to that value. Let's look at another situation. Suppose one of your values is related to building and maintaining relationships in your family. Yesterday, were there any moments where you kept to yourself or avoided communicating with a loved one? Or did you have some moments of real connection with a family member?

Considering your actions in light of your values can help you see that actually you may be living your life in a way that aligns with what's important to you. Or you might notice moments when there are certain obstacles, either in the environment or within yourself, that stop you from living in line with your values. The point of this activity is not to judge yourself, whether you are doing well or not, but simply to recognize what's in front of you and make a conscious choice to live in a more meaningful way. No one can be perfect all the time and do everything in line with their values. The important thing is to see where you are at and to keep taking small steps towards your values.

Recognising your values and aligning your actions with what truly matters to you can be a powerful way to support your mental well-being. Values are the guiding principles that reflect the kind of person you want to be and the life you want to lead, while goals are the concrete steps you take to move in that direction. By identifying your values, whether it is being a loving partner, staying active, or continuing to learn, you can create meaningful goals that give your life direction and purpose, even in the face of challenges. Reflecting on your daily activities through the lens of your values can help you see which actions bring you closer to the life you want and which take you away from it. Using tools like the SMART goal framework can make your goals more achievable. It is also important to anticipate and plan for barriers, such as Parkinson's symptoms or practical difficulties, so you can adapt your actions without losing sight of your values. Staying motivated involves taking small, consistent steps, seeking support, and reminding yourself regularly of what matters most. With clarity about your values, you can navigate the ups and downs of Parkinson's with a greater sense of meaning and direction. Although you did not choose to have Parkinson's, it is still within your power to choose what you want to do. No one says you have to take control of what you do. However, you may find that life is much more interesting and helpful when you do.

FURTHER READING

Some resources to expand on mental health and well-being in Parkinson's as well as explaining further the key acceptance and commitment therapy concepts, of being open, aware, and present.

The Happiness Trap. (n.d.). *Acceptance and commitment therapy free resources*. Retrieved June 4, 2025, from https://thehappinesstrap.com/free-resources/

Oxford Mindfulness. (n.d.). *Mindfulness resources*. Retrieved June 4, 2025, from https://oxfordmindfulness.org/events-and-resources

The PACT App. (n.d.). *Acceptance and commitment therapy for Parkinson's, free videos and audios*. Retrieved June 4, 2025, from https://www.pact.guide/

Parkinson's Foundation. (n.d.). *Emotional and mental health*. Retrieved June 4, 2025, from https://www.parkinson.org/living-with-parkinsons/emotional-mental-health

REFERENCES

Aarsland, D., Påhlhagen, S., Ballard, C. G., Ehrt, U., & Svenningsson, P. (2012). Depression in Parkinson disease – epidemiology, mechanisms and management. *Nature Reviews Neurology*, *8*(1), 35–47.

British Psychological Society. (2021). *Psychological interventions for people with Huntington's disease, Parkinson's disease, motor neurone disease, and multiple sclerosis: Evidence-based guidance*. British Psychological Society.

Candel-Parra, E., Córcoles-Jiménez, M. P., Delicado-Useros, V., Ruiz-Grao, M. C., Hernández-Martínez, A., & Molina-Alarcón, M. (2022).

Predictive model of quality of life in patients with Parkinson's disease. *International Journal of Environmental Research and Public Health*, *19*(2), 672.

Chaudhuri, K. R., & Schapira, A. H. (2009). Non-motor symptoms of Parkinson's disease: Dopaminergic pathophysiology and treatment. *The Lancet Neurology*, *8*(5), 464–474. https://doi.org/10.1016/S1474-4422(09)70068-7

Deane, K. H., Flaherty, H., Daley, D. J., Pascoe, R., Penhale, B., Clarke, C. E., Sackley, C. & Storey, S. (2014). Priority setting partnership to identify the top 10 research priorities for the management of Parkinson's disease. *BMJ open*, *4*(12), e006434.

Den Brok, M. G., van Dalen, J. W., van Gool, W. A., Moll van Charante, E. P., de Bie, R. M., & Richard, E. (2015). Apathy in Parkinson's disease: A systematic review and meta-analysis. *Movement Disorders*, *30*(6), 759–769.

Dissanayaka, N. N., Sellbach, A., Matheson, S., O'Sullivan, J. D., Silburn, P. A., Byrne, G. J., . . . & Mellick, G. D. (2010). Anxiety disorders in Parkinson's disease: Prevalence and risk factors. *Movement Disorders*, *25*(7), 838–845.

Dobkin, R. D., Interian, A., Durland, J. L., Gara, M. A., & Menza, M. A. (2018). Personalized telemedicine for depression in Parkinson's disease: A pilot trial. *Journal of Geriatric Psychiatry and Neurology*, *31*(4), 171–176.

Dobkin, R. D., Mann, S. L., Gara, M. A., Interian, A., Rodriguez, K. M., & Menza, M. (2020). Telephone-based cognitive behavioral therapy for depression in Parkinson disease: A randomized controlled trial. *Neurology*, *94*(16), e1764–e1773.

Even, C., & Weintraub, D. (2012). Is depression in Parkinson's disease (PD) a specific entity? *Journal of Affective Disorders*, *139*(2), 103–112.

Galante, J., Friedrich, C., Dawson, A. F., Modrego-Alarcón, M., Gebbing, P., Delgado-Suárez, I., Gupta, R., Dean, L., Dalgleish, T., White, I. R., & Jones, P. B. (2021). Mindfulness-based programmes for mental health promotion in adults in nonclinical settings: A systematic review and meta-analysis of randomised controlled trials. *PLOS Medicine*, *18*(1), e1003481.

Hayes, S. C. (2004). Acceptance and commitment therapy, relational frame theory, and the third wave of behavioral and cognitive therapies. *Behavior Therapy*, *35*(4), 639–665.

Hinnell, C., Hurt, C. S., Landau, S., Brown, R. G., Samuel, M., & PROMS-PD Study Group. (2012). Nonmotor versus motor symptoms: How much do they matter to health status in Parkinson's disease? *Movement Disorders*, *27*(2), 236–241.

Ishihara, L., & Brayne, C. (2006). A systematic review of depression and mental illness preceding Parkinson's disease. *Acta Neurologica Scandinavica*, *113*(4), 211–220.

Jacob, E. L., Gatto, N. M., Thompson, A., Bordelon, Y., & Ritz, B. (2010). Occurrence of depression and anxiety prior to Parkinson's disease. *Parkinsonism & Related Disorders*, *16*(9), 576–581.

Kuyken, W., Warren, F. C., Taylor, R. S., Whalley, B., Crane, C., Bondolfi, G., Hayes, R., Huijbers, M., Ma, H., Schweizer, S., Segal, Z., Speckens, A., Teasdale, J. D., Van Heeringen, K., Williams, M., Byford, S., Byng, R., & Dalgleish, T. (2016). Efficacy of mindfulness-based cognitive therapy in prevention of depressive relapse: An individual patient data meta-analysis from randomized trials. *JAMA Psychiatry*, *73*(6), 565–574.

National Institute for Health and Care Excellence. (2021). *Chronic pain (primary and secondary) in over 16s: Assessment of all chronic pain and management of chronic primary pain*. National Institute for Health and Care Excellence.

Pluck, G. C., & Brown, R. G. (2002). Apathy in Parkinson's disease. *Journal of Neurology, Neurosurgery & Psychiatry*, *73*(6), 636–642.

Reijnders, J. S., Ehrt, U., Weber, W. E., Aarsland, D., & Leentjens, A. F. (2008). A systematic review of prevalence studies of depression in Parkinson's disease. *Movement Disorders*, *23*(2), 183–189.

Simpson, J., Lekwuwa, G., & Crawford, T. (2013). Illness beliefs and psychological outcome in people with Parkinson's disease. *Chronic Illness*, *9*(2), 165–176.

Simpson, J., McMillan, H., Leroi, I., & Murray, C. D. (2014). Experiences of apathy in people with Parkinson's disease: A qualitative exploration. *Disability and Rehabilitation*, *37*(7), 611–619. https://doi.org/10.3109/0 9638288.2014.939771

Simpson, J., & Thomas, C. (2015). Clinical psychology and disability studies: Bridging the disciplinary divide on mental health and disability. *Disability and Rehabilitation*, *37*(14), 1299–1304.

Tuijt, R., Tan, A., Armstrong, M., Pigott, J., Read, J., Davies, N., Walters, K., & Schrag, A. (2020). Self-management components as experienced by people with Parkinson's disease and their carers: A systematic review and synthesis of the qualitative literature. *Parkinson's Disease*, *2020*(1), 8857385.

Weintraub, D., & Burn, D. J. (2011). Parkinson's disease: The quintessential neuropsychiatric disorder. *Movement Disorders, 26*(6), 1022–1031.

Wieringa, G., Dale, M., & Eccles, F. J. (2022). Adjusting to living with Parkinson's disease; a meta-ethnography of qualitative research. *Disability and Rehabilitation, 44*(23), 6949–6968.

Yazd, S. A. R., Gashtil, S., Moradpoor, M., Pishdar, S., Nabian, P., Kazemi, Z., & Naeim, M. (2023). Reducing depression and anxiety symptoms in patients with Parkinson's disease: The effectiveness of group cognitive behavioral therapy. *Parkinsonism & Related Disorders, 112*, 105456.

3

HOW CAN I MANAGE PARKINSON'S SYMPTOMS EFFECTIVELY?

Over the years, researchers and psychologists have been looking for what makes it easier or harder to adjust to a long-term condition. Environmental, societal, psychological, and illness factors, all play a role in your experience with the condition. However, the one factor that is consistently found to facilitate adjustment across all different long-term conditions is self-efficacy. Self-efficacy is the belief you have in your ability to handle situations, and this belief can make a significant difference in how you respond to challenges.

Psychologist Albert Bandura defined self-efficacy as 'people's judgements of their capabilities to organise and execute courses of action required to attain designated types of performances' (Bandura, 1986, p. 391). Put simply, self-efficacy is not about what you *can* do objectively, but what you *believe* you can do in a specific situation (Mills et al., 2007). This distinction is important: two people with similar abilities may behave very differently based on how confident they feel about taking action. Self-efficacy is sometimes confused with self-esteem, but these two concepts are different. As Bandura explained, 'self-efficacy is a judgment of capability; self-esteem is a judgment of self-worth'.

DOI: 10.4324/9781003484332-4

Self-efficacy became a central idea in social cognitive psychology, which views individuals as active participants in their lives, capable of making choices, setting goals, and influencing outcomes (Wyatt, 2018). Bandura (1977) argued that these beliefs affect the activities we choose, the effort we put in, and how long we persist, especially when things get tough.

But how are self-efficacy beliefs formed? Bandura (1977, 1997) identified four key sources that shape our self-efficacy. First, we have the mastery experiences. These are based on your own past successes. If you have handled a similar challenge before, you are more likely to feel confident facing it again. Second, vicarious experiences. Seeing or hearing about how others, especially people in similar situations, have succeeded can boost your own confidence. This is why support groups and peer stories can be so empowering. Third factor that influences our self-efficacy beliefs is verbal persuasion. Encouragement and feedback from others, whether from family, friends, or healthcare professionals, can influence your belief in yourself. Finally, physiological and emotional states can shape our self-efficacy beliefs. How we interpret our physical and emotional state also matters. Feeling anxious, fatigued, or unwell might lower your self-belief, while feeling calm or in control can strengthen it and studies have shown that this is especially true for people with Parkinson's (Estrada-Bellmann et al., 2021). Understanding these sources can help you reflect on why you feel confident or uncertain, about certain tasks, and how you might boost your belief in your ability to manage daily life with Parkinson's.

Research has shown that self-efficacy plays a powerful role in motivation, learning, and achievement. In Parkinson's, it has shown that self-efficacy can impact motor, non-motor symptoms, and quality of life (Estrada-Bellmann et al., 2021). People who believe they can succeed are more likely to try, persist when faced with difficulties, and feel more satisfied with their progress. Interestingly, the most beneficial self-beliefs are often those that slightly overestimate one's true abilities, a small boost in confidence can help increase persistence during hard times (Artino, 2012). However, balance is key:

an overly inflated sense of confidence might lead to risky decisions or reduced effort, while too little belief can cause avoidance, frustration, and a negative impact on mental well-being.

The same logic applies to living well with Parkinson's. Believing you can manage your medications, attend an event, or complete an exercise class, even if it takes more planning or support, can improve your quality of life. On the other hand, consistently doubting your ability to cope may cause you to withdraw, miss opportunities, or feel overwhelmed. To take active steps to manage Parkinson's symptoms and your well-being, you need to believe you are capable of doing this. When I am talking about managing Parkinson's, I mean tasks that will help to control symptoms and improve well-being. Things like correct medication use, exercise, healthy eating, stress management, modified personal care, adjustment to new social and financial circumstances, pertinent communication with doctors, family members and carers, modification of your living and working environment as well as valued activities.

But let's put the theories and the evidence in practice now. Let's think back to the factors that contribute to our self-efficacy beliefs: **mastery** experiences (building a portfolio of proof that you have the skills required to succeed), **vicarious experiences** (seeing others achieving things you want to achieve and being inspired by their example), and **verbal persuasion** (having other encouraging you and giving you positive feedback as well as cultivating an inner voice that is more encouraging and less self-critical). All these will help you cultivate beliefs of capability that will then lead to improved mental health and the improved mental health will help you maintain those beliefs and you create a virtuous circle for yourself. For example, maybe you've fallen in the past and now you need to build up your confidence and walk to the shops on your own. You might want to build your confidence gradually by practicing walking in a safe supportive environment (skills **mastery)**. Maybe you can also learn by observing others with Parkinson's either in a local Parkinson's groups or online, watch people with Parkinson's who had successfully increased their activity levels (**vicarious experience**), watching others doing the thing you want to do can make you think, 'If they can do it, maybe I can too'. You can talk to you family, friends, or doctors about what you want to do and they can also provide support, motivation, and encouragement, by reminding you things you have achieved, sharing other success stories, or relevant written material (**verbal persuasion**).

If you want to increase your self-efficacy, you could set up a similar setting for yourself. First, decide on a new action that will help with your symptoms or your well-being. It could be regular exercise, medication management, or voice therapy. You can discuss this with someone close to you or a healthcare professional to help you set a meaningful and realistic goal. Then you can make a personal plan and commit to it in writing. You could share the plan with someone you feel will be able to give you feedback and encourage your progress. Or maybe you could decide to send yourself voice notes or log in a diary your small successes to keep the momentum and be able to look back at how far you have come. It could also be useful to make a list of potential setbacks or bad days. It is important to recognise both internal and external influences, like past experiences or lack of resources, that may affect motivation. You could also problem-solve together with a significant other or a healthcare professional to remove barriers (e.g. fatigue, mobility, medication side effects). You could also tap into the vicarious mastery, by talking to other people with Parkinson's and finding more about their journey, this might help you map out stages or goals you would also like to achieve. In this chapter, I will discuss ways you can manage some common Parkinson's symptoms, so you can even pick one of those symptoms or ways to address them and make your plan.

When you start setting goals, trying out new skills, sharing ideas, and offering mutual support, you start building slowly but steadily your confidence. It is also important to acknowledge that confidence does not always grow in a straight line. If past experiences with exercise or treatment were frustrating or painful, those feelings can still affect your willingness to try again. But remember, you can still grow, while you are grieving. Health professionals can support you by talking through those experiences and helping you build a step-by-step plan to regain trust in your own abilities.

It is not just your confidence. Care-partners' confidence also plays a key role. A study by Keefe et al. (2003) found that care partners who felt confident in helping a loved one manage pain, they experienced less stress, more positive mood, and reported that their loved one had better physical well-being, more energy, and fewer days spent resting in bed.

Having said all that, I also need to underline that it is not all on you, social support can play a huge role in your self-efficacy. For many years, managing long-term health conditions was seen mainly as an individual responsibility, something that depended on your own knowledge, motivation, and ability to self-manage. While those personal skills are still important, research increasingly shows that you do not have to do it alone. In fact, the support of your social network, family, friends, neighbours, fellow patients, and even colleagues can make a real difference in how well you manage life with Parkinson's. That's your 'network of networks', a personal community of people who are involved in different ways, some closely and others more loosely (Vassilev et al., 2011). These connections can provide not only practical help but also emotional encouragement, shared experiences, and a sense of belonging.

But the real power of social connection goes even further. It is not just about receiving help, it is about what happens collectively when people support one another. This is called collective efficacy, the shared belief that *together*, a group can achieve a goal (Bandura, 1986). Rather than focusing only on what one person can do alone (individual self-efficacy), collective efficacy recognises that people living with Parkinson's often lean on and lift up one another. Whether it is a group making a plan to exercise regularly, friends encouraging each other to stay positive, or family members rallying to help with appointments and routines, these are examples of coordinated, ongoing effort that make management of Parkinson's more sustainable (Vassilev et al., 2014).

Importantly, collective efficacy is not just the sum of everyone's individual confidence. It is a unique strength that emerges from how people work together, share tasks, and adapt over time. Even weaker social ties, like a neighbour who checks in occasionally or a volunteer at a Parkinson's local group, can become part of this web of support, as long as there's trust, communication, and shared purpose. In daily life, this might involve decisions like who to call for help, how to ask for support in a way that feels comfortable or even choosing not to rely too heavily on one person to avoid straining relationships. These are real and valid concerns, and learning how to navigate them is part of the ongoing 'relational work' that supports collective success.

Researchers have found that collective efficacy thrives when there is regular interaction, shared goals (even small ones), and a willingness to adapt to each other's needs. For example, in a local Parkinson's support group, members might differ in what they want, some want exercise tips, others need emotional support, but through mutual respect and conversation, they shape the group to meet everyone's needs. This kind of flexible, evolving support system helps people not just manage Parkinson's, but live well with it. So, while Parkinson's is something you live with personally, the journey is best travelled with others. Tapping into your networks, and recognising their collective strength, can help you stay motivated, resilient, and more connected.

Self-efficacy is the belief in your ability to take action and handle specific situations, and it plays a powerful role in how you manage life with Parkinson's. It is not just about what you can do, but what you believe you can do, and this belief shapes your motivation, persistence, and well-being. Confidence comes from several sources: your past successes (mastery), seeing others succeed (vicarious experience), encouragement from others (verbal persuasion), and how you interpret your emotional or physical state. Building self-efficacy through small wins, support from peers and professionals, and setting achievable goals can help you feel more in control and engaged in managing Parkinson's. People around you play an important role in helping to manage the condition, but more importantly, can be a huge source of joy or stress. Let's start by looking at communication.

3.1 HOW CAN I MANAGE COMMUNICATION DIFFICULTIES?

Communication connects us to others, helps us express who we are, and plays a central role in our relationships and sense of identity. Better understanding communication difficulties and seeking out support can have tangible benefits but also could enrich your relationships with others. Parkinson's motor symptoms and changes in voice, thinking, and energy can contribute to communication difficulties. Family members and care partners usually find ways to support the communication. This chapter explores the ways communication is affected in Parkinson's, the emotional and relational impact, and practical strategies to stay connected.

One of the most noticeable changes in communication is dysarthria, a motor speech disorder that results from the muscle rigidity and bradykinesia (slowness of movement) associated with Parkinson's. Common features include reduced voice volume (hypophonia), slurred or mumbled speech, increased pauses during speech, and variability in speech rate. These changes can make it hard for you to hear or understand, especially in group conversations or noisy environments.

Cognition also plays a big role in how we communicate. You may experience difficulty finding words, processing what other are saying or you have trouble initiating or sustaining your speech. Maybe you have trouble staying focused on others speaking for a long period of time or get easily distracted. These cognitive shifts can lead to shorter conversations, off-topic comments, or trouble keeping up with fast-paced discussions.

Embarrassment, anxiety, or fatigue can also get in the way of speaking. Many people feel self-conscious when their voice changes or when they struggle to find words. Over time, some may withdraw from social situations, which only deepens feelings of isolation and loss (Saldert & Bauer, 2017).

These changes can make talking with others more frustrating, for both you and the people close to you. Some people with Parkinson's say they feel like they're not being heard or understood. Others say they avoid conversations altogether because it takes too much energy or because they're worried about being judged.

Changes in communication often feel like personal losses. You may grieve the ability to tell jokes, lead conversations, or participate in activities you once loved. Family members may feel the absence of shared conversations and spontaneous connection. Studies have shown that families respond in many ways, some accept the new reality, other find seeking information to understand and cope helpful, a lot of families normalise the changes within the family and show empathy and patience, which become essential emotional tools. Recognising these emotional responses is a step towards compassion for everyone involved.

Some people find that long-standing communication patterns with a partner or family member do not work as well anymore, which can lead to misunderstandings or hurt feelings. But recognising these changes is the first step to finding new ways to connect. If you're struggling, let your loved ones know. They may not realise what you're experiencing unless you share it.

Common repair strategies used by partners include reminding, prompting, repeating, or guessing what was said, asking for clarification, offering suggested words, helping steer the topic back on course, initiating new topics when needed. You might find some of these strategies helpful and others less so. It is important to have an honest conversation with your partner about things that help or do not help. You could even have a notebook that you note those down for your partner to read. Involving your significant others can bring you closer together and people generally appreciate when they feel helpful.

There are a few things that can help, for example, if both you and your conversation partner speak slowly, enunciate your words, and give each other time to speak and respond can improve speech clarity and comprehension. Using short, simple sentences and pausing between phrases can also enhance understanding. External/environmental factors can also help, for example, sitting face-to-face or next to each other can help improve understanding, turning off the TV or moving to a quieter space when having a conversation can also help. If fatigue gets in the way of communication, remember, you don't always have to be the talker. Some people with Parkinson's find it comforting to take on more of a listening role when they're tired. Being part of the conversation doesn't always mean speaking, it can also mean simply being present and enjoying the connection. Practice active listening by maintaining eye contact, nodding in acknowledgement, and paraphrasing or summarising key points to ensure understanding and demonstrate engagement in the conversation. If reduced facial expressions is the issue for you then maybe incorporating visual aids such as gesture cues could help.

Speech therapists can help you strengthen your voice and teach strategies to improve communication. Talking to a speech and language therapist could also provide you with tailor practical speech tips you could use and how to go about using those, they might, for example, be able to suggest amplification devices or voice training programmes. Speech therapies could also take a more holistic view of the issues and suggest other strategies to do with how you structure your environment, creating routines and using written notes and visual aids.

3.2 HOW TO MANAGE MILD COGNITIVE DIFFICULTIES?

Sometimes my brain 'freezes up,' kind of like my legs sometimes do. Finding the words I want to say is very hard, and my thoughts seem like they are blank.

(Goldman et al., 2018)

Maybe you had a similar experience. Forgetting words, our thread of thoughts, or why we enter a room is not unusual and some cognitive lapses will happen as we get old. However, these issues might also be part of Parkinson's manifestation; in fact, mild cognitive impairment prevalence is estimated around 40% of people with Parkinson's. Mild cognitive impairment means that you might feel distracted or disorganised, along with finding it difficult to plan and accomplish tasks. It may be harder to focus in situations that divide your attention, like a group conversation. When facing a task or situation on your own, you may feel overwhelmed by having to make choices. You may also have difficulty remembering information or have trouble finding the right words when speaking. These changes can range from being annoying to interfering with managing household affairs (Parkinson's Foundation, 2025a).

A question frequently expressed by people living with Parkinson's is whether the cognitive changes they notice are part of 'ageing' or because of Parkinson's. In 'normal' ageing, cognitive problems typically involve difficulty with recalling and generating words or names (tip of the tongue phenomenon). Forgetting words and names is also common in Parkinson's. Cognitive difficulties can occur as we age and as neuropathways and brain activity changes. Parkinson's-related mild cognitive impairment primarily affects memory, visuo-spatial (understanding and manipulating visual information, solving puzzles and following directions), and executive functions (goal-directed behaviours processed by the frontal lobes of the brain (Aciyiyen, 2023). In general, cognitive changes in 'normal' ageing should not interfere significantly with everyday activities that require cognitive abilities. If they do, however, this may suggest that might be what we call mild cognitive impairment. Changes in functional abilities and everyday activities due to cognitive decline can be difficult to identify if they are mild. Distinguishing whether problems in everyday activities are due to cognitive or motor problems in Parkinson's, or a combination of both, can also be challenging. Disentangling effects of age-related and disease-related changes on cognition, non-motor issues (e.g. sleep disturbances, mood disorders, apathy, and fatigue), and medications is difficult.

Research has shown mild cognitive impairment is associated with older age, lower education, longer disease duration, higher levodopa equivalent daily dose, more severe motor symptoms, and postural instability/gait difficulty motor subtype, poorer quality of life, hallucinations, higher levels of apathy, and depression (Baiano et al., 2020). Mild cognitive impairment has also been identified as a risk factor for the development of dementia (Caviness et al., 2007; Williams-Gray et al., 2009) but that is not always the case (Williams-Gray et al., 2007).

There are pharmacological and non-pharmacological approaches to address cognitive impairments but here I will focus on non-pharmacological approaches, especially those that we have evidence of being helpful (i.e. physical activity; brain stimulation) rather than those with less evidence in Parkinson's (i.e. cognitive training, cognitive rehabilitation, nutrition).

There is growing evidence that physical exercise may benefit cognitive function, particularly in the early to moderate stages of Parkinson's. Exercise may influence the brain through increased dopamine signalling, stimulation of neurotrophic factors (which support neuron health), improved blood flow, and changes in brain structure and function, especially in areas like the prefrontal cortex, which plays a key role in executive function. Various types of exercise, including aerobic, resistance, and dance can improve cognitive function, although the optimal type, amount, mechanisms, and duration of exercise are unclear (Murray et al., 2014). We also do not know whether there are other factors that make exercising harder and these factors (e.g. social isolation) increase cognitive difficulties rather than the protective effects of exercise. Importantly, exercise might not only help cognition directly but also indirectly, by reducing depression, improving sleep, and increasing social engagement, all of which can positively influence brain function.

Different types of exercises have been explored. Aerobic exercises like walking and cycling appear to boost executive function. A major review of 29 randomised controlled trials involving over

2,000 older adults found that engaging in aerobic activity, typically three times per week at moderate intensity for several months, led to improvements in mental processing speed, memory, and executive functions like planning and decision-making. These benefits were particularly noticeable when people exercised at least 150 minutes per week and were maintained up to 18 months after the exercise programmes ended. Some of these studies also showed improvements in depression scores, motor function, and quality of life. Progressive resistance training (strengthening exercises) and general strength programmes can also help with improved working memory and executive function. Multi-modal exercise programmes, combining aerobic activity, strength training, flexibility, and balance, have also shown cognitive benefits. Even less conventional forms of physical activity, like Argentine tango dancing, have demonstrated cognitive benefits. Tango, in particular, has been associated with improvements in spatial cognition, although results for overall cognitive improvement have been mixed. Finally, mind body exercises, such as Tai Chi, Qigong, and yoga, can be recommended strategies for improving cognitive function in people with cognitive impairment and Parkinson's.

While we do not yet have a one-size-fits-all prescription, there's strong reason to include regular physical activity as part of a holistic approach to managing Parkinson's, especially for those with mild cognitive impairment or concerns about thinking skills.

Transcranial magnetic stimulation (TMS) is a non-invasive treatment that uses magnetic pulses to stimulate specific areas of the brain. Repetitive TMS has been studied for improving movement, mood, and thinking skills in Parkinson's. While some early studies suggest it might help with cognition, the evidence so far is mixed.

Another similar method being studied is transcranial direct current stimulation (tDCS), which uses a mild electrical current to activate certain brain regions. Some studies have shown that tDCS, especially when applied to the front part of the brain (called the dorsolateral prefrontal cortex), can improve aspects of thinking such as attention, working memory, and verbal fluency in people with

Parkinson's. However, we still do not have strong evidence for its effectiveness but some indications that it can help improve verbal fluency.

Overall, studies of brain stimulation in Parkinson's show mixed results. Some people may experience improvements in specific thinking skills, especially when treatments are combined with cognitive or physical training, but not everyone responds the same way. These treatments also require regular visits and trained professionals, which may be time-consuming or tiring for some. As research continues, we'll hopefully learn more about who is most likely to benefit and how to tailor these treatments for each individual.

Mild cognitive impairment in Parkinson's is linked to factors like older age, longer disease duration, higher medication doses, and worse motor symptoms. Mild cognitive impairment raises the risk for dementia (a severe loss of intellectual abilities) but doesn't always lead to it. Non-pharmacological strategies, especially exercise, are emerging as effective ways to support cognitive function. Brain stimulation may also help, but more research is needed to tailor these methods to individual needs. Tell your doctor if you have concerns about cognitive changes. You may need to change your medication or see a neurologist or neuropsychologist for assessment. An occupational therapist can also help you find strategies for adapting and coping with these symptoms. A speech therapist can help with language difficulties.

3.3 HOW TO MANAGE PAIN?

About 7.8 million people live with chronic pain. Pain is a common symptom shared among many people with long-term conditions. I have written about pain and how to manage it in my previous book on *Living Well with a Long-Term Health Condition* (Bogosian, 2020), here, I will revisit some of the main principles but also tailor the advice to what is most relevant in Parkinson's.

In Parkinson's, pain can be related to a number of issues. It could be musculoskeletal pain due to Parkinson's affecting the bones, muscles, ligaments, tendons, and nerves. It can occur suddenly or be long-lasting and can occur in one area or several. People might also experience neuropathic/radicular pain due to damage to nerves occurring anywhere from where the fibres leave the spinal cord to where they end in the skin. Dystonic pain is from sustained or repetitive muscle twisting, spasm, or cramp that can occur at different times of day and in different stages of Parkinson's. Rigidity, weakened muscles, and involuntary muscle contractions (dystonia) can cause painful deformities for people with Parkinson's (Parkinson's Foundation, 2025c). Akathisia, the feeling of restlessness or inability to be still, is also a form of pain that can be experienced in Parkinson's. Finally, central pain is pain due to the pathways which control sensation and pain in the brain, brainstem, and spinal cord not working properly (Parkinson's Foundation, 2025c). To help your doctor figure out the cause of the pain take some mental, written, or voice notes on where the pain is located, whether it stays or moves around, what does the pain feel like, whether it is continuous or comes and goes, anything that might be triggering the pain or whether specific times of the day the pain gets better or worse. It would be also useful to note down anything that relieves your pain or makes it worse.

It is not surprising that the pain is closely related to other symptoms, mobility limitations, depression, anxiety, and sleep disturbances. Consequently, these other symptoms can lead to avoidance behaviour, unhelpful thoughts and beliefs, and emotional difficulties. In turn, these behaviours, thoughts, and emotions can lead back to increased pain. For example, pain keeps you awake at night, and because you can't sleep, you keep looking at the clock, thinking that with this restless night you won't be able to function properly the next day, and you start feeling anxious, which makes it harder to fall asleep by being so worked up, and then poor sleep by itself or in combination with all the other thoughts, emotions, and behaviour patterns can make pain worse. Stress, anxiety, and emotions such as depression, anger, fear, and frustration are all normal responses to living with a long-term condition, like Parkinson's, and they can increase your pain and discomfort. When you are stressed, angry, afraid, or depressed, everything, including your pain, seems worse.

What does it mean to manage your pain? Surely, the point must be to rid yourself of the pain and not 'manage' it. A lot of people with a long-term condition have 'managing pain' high on their agenda. Living with unending pain can play havoc with any plans of spending your time meaningfully and with intention. We humans are active problem-solving agents. The misdirected problem-solving drive can sometimes be a mission impossible, an insoluble problem. Although eliminating the pain might not be feasible for a lot of people, finding ways to gain some control over the pain so it is less overwhelming might be a more realistic goal.

Research evidence demonstrates that there isn't much correlation between changes in pain and other psychological outcome and numerous studies have shown that very good treatment outcomes can be achieved without pain reduction. If pain cannot effectively be reduced, the content of the thoughts and beliefs about pain appears to be a good place to start working.

Avoiding activities because of the pain can ultimately lead to more pain. The way we can combat this naturally occurring avoidance when it comes to pain is by accepting that pain is part of your condition. Avoiding activities can lead to disuse, disability, and depression that can exacerbate the pain.

On the other hand, you might want to carry on everything you used to do despite being in pain. You have some ideas of how things should be and you want to get back to what you consider your normal life disregarding any signals from your body. In some case though, this perseverance can lead to frustration, distress, hypervigilance, and further disability.

The toughest challenge when it comes to managing your pain and most of the symptoms is to battle your own mind. It is true your mind loves you and will never hurt you but also your mind wants to take short cuts and worries far too much about the future. So, how do you win against your mind? Simply by recognising its tricks, acknowledging that they are only tricks and letting them go.

You might have thoughts like 'If I wake up feeling pain my day is ruined', or 'If I ask my colleagues to reschedule the meeting, they'll think I'm not pulling my weight' or 'Nothing has worked to help me with the pain, so these techniques won't help either'. These thoughts are lies we tell ourselves; the truth is far less harsh – having pain does not necessarily mean your whole day is ruined, your colleagues won't think that you are not pulling your weight because you reschedule a meeting and just because you haven't found something to help you with the pain so far does not mean that managing your pain through controlling your thoughts will not help either.

Think back to the last time you had pain. What unhelpful thought did you have? If that thought comes back again, you can recognise it for what it is and it will be less likely that you will engage with it and let it ruin your mood or your plans.

Hassan has early-onset Parkinson's disease, and although he does not experience many Parkinson's symptoms, he frequently gets intense pain in his shoulder and stiffness in his neck. Pain relief medication did not offer much relief. Hassan's main coping strategy was to distract himself with video games.

However, distraction and videogames did not always help. It was difficult for him to concentrate on other activities when in pain. He decided to join our mindfulness course. One of the exercises we did in the course was to focus on the pain and explore the physical sensation of the pain. Where is the pain? Does it move around or stay in the same place? Does pain intensity change? How does the pain feel, burning, stabbing, stinging, etc.? The idea was that without judging or qualifying the pain to stay with it and explore it with kindness and curiosity.

Naturally, Hassan hated this mindfulness practice. Who wouldn't? He said the pain was getting worse and worse as he was focusing on it. Despite how much he disliked the practice, he agreed to experiment with it again in the next sessions. When at home, watching TV worked most of the time as a distraction from the pain, but he wanted to try something different for the times when not even TV could distract him. In the fourth session, he observed that when noticing the pain, his mind played out all sorts of unpleasant scenarios, about how bad this is, that the pain is debilitating, that he can't go on suffering like that. It happened very quickly, his mind flicking between noticing the pain and having thoughts about the 'badness' of the situation. That was his breakthrough. He saw how the mind was intruding and making things worse. The pain was present, and he could do very little about it, but he could let the thoughts about pain go.

After Hassan noticed his thoughts and started practicing letting them go without identifying with them too much. As well as the pain, I asked him to notice other things, for example, his breath and the fact that he is breathing or the sounds around him. By the end of the 8-week course, Hassan was able to widen and narrow his attentional focus while staying with the painful sensation. Being able to focus on other things without ignoring the pain opened up more choices and gave him more freedom. He can now choose what he wants to do, not just do the things that will distract him from pain.

Being aware of your thoughts, emotions, and coping mechanisms and their potential effects on your pain level is a good start in your pain management journey. Staying connected to your personal values and goals can help you disengage from these unhelpful thoughts.

By accepting the pain, it is less likely that you will try to avoid thoughts around pain or avoid engaging in physical activity or other activities you value. Research has also shown that diverting attention away from painful stimuli can be unhelpful.

Watching TV, exercising, reading, or engaging in other pleasant non-demanding activities could help distract from the pain. When reducing the pain or getting rid of the pain is beyond our control, distraction might be the most beneficial way to cope with the pain. There are situations though that distraction is not as helpful. Hassan sometimes did not want to watch TV, he wanted to cook dinner or play with his kids, but doing anything physical reminded him of his shoulder pain and was not a sufficient distraction. Staying with the pain in this more accepting and open way gave him the options to do other things in the evenings. By accepting the pain, we eliminate a layer of suffering (the unpleasant thoughts that usually accompany the pain), and also instead of spending time and energy ignoring the pain, we let the pain be while directing our attention to whatever we intend to do.

3.4 HOW TO MANAGE FATIGUE?

Do you ever feel like sometimes you just wake up on the wrong side of the bed and all of a sudden you're having the hardest day ever, especially with 'off' fluctuations, your body is completely exhausted you have no energy to do anything you can't think straight and you're just in a rut. This could be fatigue. In this section, I will discuss some ideas to manage fatigue that I had also discussed in my previous book (Bogosian, 2020). Here, I will expand those ideas and discuss them within the context of Parkinson's.

About half of the people with Parkinson's report that fatigue is a major problem, and one-third say it is their most disabling symptom. As someone with Parkinson's once told me, 'it's like two 3-year-olds hanging around each leg all day long'. The impact of fatigue can be severe. Extreme exhaustion that comes with fatigue can lead people to avoid social activities, reduce hours at work, or even retire. Understanding fatigue and finding ways to cope with it are essential to maintaining a good quality of life (Parkinson's Foundation, 2025b). Here, we will explore some ways to deal with the difficult days. Ways that don't involve spending time wishing things were different, indulging in habits that push us further away from our goals or neglecting ourselves and the people we care about.

Fatigue is a common early symptom in the course of Parkinson's, but can occur at any point and can happen whether movement symptoms are mild or severe. Fatigue can occur on its own or along with other symptoms such as sleep disturbances, pain, or depression. Stress can make fatigue worse. The cause of fatigue in Parkinson's is unknown. It is possible that motor symptoms like tremor and stiffness contribute to making muscles tired, but because fatigue occurs even in those with mild motor symptoms, this is probably not the only explanation. It is important to consider that fatigue can have causes outside of Parkinson's and to identify illnesses or medications unrelated to Parkinson's that may contribute to fatigue.

Sometimes pressure, strain, and stress can also be confused with fatigue. If you feel under pressure, the strain will increase the likelihood that the pressure turns into stress and stress can often lead to exacerbation of fatigue. By learning to discern between fatigue, strain, pressure, and stress, you naturally increase your capacity to handle fatigue skilfully. For example, if you see that you're on the verge of strain, you might decide not to do certain things that would push you over. A lot of the times, even when we are doing enough, we might feel that we haven't achieved much. Keeping a log of small daily wins or achievements at the end of each day or even starting the day with a list of things you achieved the previous day instead of a standard to-do list will help boost your confidence and reduce your stress, which can contribute to fatigue.

Figuring out what exacerbates fatigue can help you find the best way to combat it. Inactivity is a common cause of fatigue in long-term conditions. Muscles that are not used become de-conditioned and less efficient at doing what they are supposed to do. Poor nutrition can be another reason. Food that is inferior quality or not consumed in the appropriate quantities will not give the body the appropriate fuel to work. Sleep difficulties can also lead to increased feelings of fatigue.

Having all or nothing type of behavioural patterns can also add to experiencing fatigue. Commonly, on the days people have more energy they try to cram in everything they can. And as you can imagine, this leads to energy crashing. Even though you feel you are achieving a lot during the 'good' days, following the intense activity you're left feeling lethargic and depleted. To increase the amount of stuff you can achieve despite your fatigue is to practice pacing. Start by doing things that you can comfortably manage without exerting yourself and build up from there slowly. The key word here is consistency. Plan to do a little but every day.

To begin with, work out your starting point, what you can manage comfortably now. To 'pace-up' an activity you should plan to do a bit more each day or every second day. Each increase should be small, and you should not do more than you planned, even if you feel like it. It also helps if you break up larger tasks into smaller steps. Create a list of all the smaller steps and based on how much you can manage now and your 'pace-up' rate create a rough timeline of completion. Recording your progress can be very motivating. It is also essential to take frequent, quick breaks. Do something for a set amount of time – 15 minutes is a good length of time – then take a break – then do a bit more – then take another brief break – and so on.

Cognitive behavioural therapy, graded exercise, mindfulness training, and sleep and stress management can improve symptoms of fatigue, however research evidence focusing specifically in Parkinson's are sparse. In cognitive behavioural therapy, you will be working with your therapist identifying unhelpful thoughts and finding ways to modify these thoughts, so they won't hold you back. Graded exercise involves physical activity that increases in intensity. Mindfulness training is based on daily meditation practices that aim to increase your present moment awareness, acceptance, and self-compassion. You can read more about sleep and stress management training, including techniques, in Chapter 4.

A common ingredient that is included in these interventions is working on fear avoidance of beliefs and behaviours. Repetitive thoughts and emotions like fear and anger can fatigue the mind and avoiding physical movement can further fatigue the body.

To summarise, things you can do to help manage your fatigue include finding out what exacerbates the fatigue, like stress, sleep, exercise and nutrition and minimise their impact. Further, look into your all-or-nothing behaviours and try to avoid the 'catching-up-on-all-the-things-when-you-can' trap. Avoid over-scheduling and learn to say no to added responsibilities or tasks you don't enjoy, you could also delegate or hire help for tasks you find particularly stressful and tiring. It can also be a good idea to plan highest levels of activity for times when you are rested and your medications are working well.

3.5 HOW CAN YOU COMMUNICATE BEST WITH HEALTHCARE PROFESSIONALS?

Access to healthcare services for people with Parkinson's is not always easy. Studies have reported delays in diagnosis, a lack of appropriate healthcare services, especially in underserved regions, and extensive waiting lists for specialist services. However, there is one thing that you can control to get the support you would like, and that is your ability to communicate clearly your needs and ask confidently for further information that will help you to make decisions. I don't mean briefly explaining issues with side effects, I mean being able to seek help for all types of symptoms you are experiencing, openly discussing them and asking for advice, guidance, and further referrals. And yes, of course, doctors and other health professionals always seem busy, sometimes do not ask open questions and you might feel they are not interested in knowing more or you are not confident they know enough to help you. But if you allow me to generalise for a minute, doctors and other health professionals have chosen those careers because they want to help people, and mostly they want to help in a way that is kind and compassionate. There is power in mastering communication with your medical team. Effective communication ensures personalised and comprehensive care. Here we will look at ways to improve this communication.

Communication in healthcare is a two-way process between you and the healthcare provider. Studies reported the breakdowns of communication could happen from either side of this relationship (Zaman et al., 2021). Nonetheless, the healthcare professionals should achieve the necessary communication skills through the training they attend before they enter practice; the opportunity to improve the communication skills of patients is scarce by comparison. For instance, some people with Parkinson's do not access mental health support because they lack understanding of their mental health, and the health professionals fail to screen them and refer them appropriately (Dobkin et al., 2013). Similarly, in a Canadian study, people with Parkinson's and their care-partners reported not receiving appropriate information or support from the health care system around palliative care (Giles & Miyasaki, 2009).

A prospective study interviewing partner-carers emphasised the importance of engaging and educating partners to promote patient-centred care (Rastgardani et al., 2019). Inconsistent and insufficient information from physicians resulted in anxiety and insecurity for partner-carers (Giles & Miyasaki, 2009). Therefore, sufficient information about the disease provided by healthcare professionals, understanding and assistance from others in public places, and psychological support for care partners might reduce their burden and improve the quality of life.

Adequate communication with doctors leads to reinforcement of medication information, psychological support, effective problem-solving, and satisfaction. It is comforting when doctors explain in detail the disease and medications, as well as dosage adjustments that addressed fears of dementia and physical discomfort. Some people completely follow their doctors' instructions based on absolute trust and others don't. A lack of education and information regarding Parkinson's provided by healthcare professionals and insufficient emotional support can lead to dissatisfaction (Boersma et al., 2016).

Due to limited time during the clinic visit, you may feel rushed and not get the information and involvement you would like (Schrag et al., 2018). It could help to have prepared your questions and what you want to share in advance to ensure that all relevant issues are addressed during your appointment. Therefore, helping doctors to understand your needs and acquire appropriate, timely solutions or adequate educational materials will make you feel better about your treatment. Next time you visit a health professional don't forget to draft questions, the questions could be about your symptoms, changes you have noticed, your medication, potential side effects, suggestions for referrals to physiotherapists, speech and language therapists or psychologists.

Self-monitoring techniques can help you gather good information about your symptoms and how they change that you can then discuss with your neurologist, Parkinson's nurse or your GP. A very simple technique is keeping a diary to record fluctuations in mood or Parkinson's symptoms with dates and times. Once you have observed the symptoms it is also important to transparently communicate your symptoms to healthcare professionals, as well as whether and how often you do end up taking your medications, and any lifestyle habits enables healthcare providers to tailor support and advice to suit your needs and preferences. Engage in shared decision-making with healthcare providers, actively participating in treatment planning and goal setting can promote mutual understanding and partnership in care planning and delivery.

It is important to be honest with your care team so they can help manage symptoms and suggest coping strategies. Discuss mood changes with your doctor so that all care decisions can be made with as much information as possible. Everyone, not only people with Parkinson's, should bring a companion to important medical appointments for support, to take notes, ask questions, and share information.

FURTHER READING

Here are some resources that expand on the management of common Parkinson's non-motor symptoms.

Bogosian, A. (2020). *Living well with a long-term health condition: An evidence-based guide to managing your symptoms*. Routledge.

The British Pain Society. (n.d.). *Understanding pain*. Retrieved June 4, 2025, from https://www.britishpainsociety.org/static/uploads/resources/files/book_understanding_pain.pdf

Jordan, M. (2020). *Coping with mild cognitive impairment (MCI): A guide to managing memory loss, effective brain training and reducing the risk of dementia.* Jessica Kingsley Publishers.

Parkinson's Foundation. (n.d.). *What can I do to improve speech and communication.* Retrieved June 4, 2025, from https://www.parkinson.org/blog/tips/speech-communication

REFERENCES

Aciyiyen, E. (2023). *Characterization of mild cognitive impairment in Parkinson's disease.* [Master's Degree Dissertation, University of Padova]. Padua Thesis and Dissertation Archive.

Artino, A. R. (2012). Academic self-efficacy: From educational theory to instructional practice. *Perspectives on Medical Education, 1,* 76–85.

Baiano, C., Barone, P., Trojano, L., & Santangelo, G. (2020). Prevalence and clinical aspects of mild cognitive impairment in Parkinson's disease: A meta-analysis. *Movement Disorders, 35*(1), 45–54.

Bandura, A. (1977). Self-efficacy: Toward a unifying theory of behavioral change. *Psychological Review, 84*(2), 191.

Bandura, A. (1986). *Social foundations of thought and action: A social cognitive theory.* Prentice-Hall.

Bandura, A. (1997). *Self-efficacy.* W. H. Freeman and Co.

Boersma, I., Jones, J., Carter, J., Bekelman, D., Miyasaki, J., Kutner, J., & Kluger, B. (2016). Parkinson disease patients' perspectives on palliative care needs: What are they telling us? *Neurology: Clinical Practice, 6*(3), 209–219.

Bogosian, A. (2020). *Living well with a long-term health condition: An evidence-based guide to managing your symptoms.* Routledge.

Caviness, J. N., Driver-Dunckley, E., Connor, D. J., Sabbagh, M. N., Hentz, J. G., Noble, B., Evidente, V. G. H., Shill, H. A., & Adler, C. H. (2007). Defining mild cognitive impairment in Parkinson's disease. *Movement Disorders: Official Journal of the Movement Disorder Society, 22*(9), 1272–1277.

Dobkin, R. D., Rubino, J. T., Friedman, J., Allen, L. A., Gara, M. A., & Menza, M. (2013). Barriers to mental health care utilization in Parkinson's disease. *Journal of Geriatric Psychiatry and Neurology, 26*(2), 105–116.

Estrada-Bellmann, I., Meléndez-Flores, J. D., Cámara-Lemarroy, C. R., & Castillo-Torres, S. A. (2021). Determinants of self-efficacy in patients with Parkinson's disease. *Arquivos de Neuro-Psiquiatria, 79*(8), 686–691.

Giles, S., & Miyasaki, J. (2009). Palliative stage Parkinson's disease: Patient and family experiences of health-care services. *Palliative Medicine, 23*(2), 120–125.

Goldman, J. G., Vernaleo, B. A., Camicioli, R., Dahodwala, N., Dobkin, R. D., Ellis, T., Galvin, J. E., Marras, C., Edwards, J., Fields, J., Golden, R., Karlawish, J., Levin, B., Shulman, L., Smith, G., Tangney, C., Thomas, C. A., Tröster, A, I., Uc, E. Y., Coyan, N., Ellman, C., . . . Simmonds, D. (2018). Cognitive impairment in Parkinson's disease: A report from a multidisciplinary symposium on unmet needs and future directions to maintain cognitive health. *npj Parkinson's Disease, 4*(1), 19.

Keefe, F. J., Ahles, T. A., Porter, L. S., Sutton, L. M., McBride, C. M., Pope, M. S., McKinstry, E. T., Furstenberg, C. P., Dalton, J., & Baucom, D. H. (2003). The self-efficacy of family caregivers for helping cancer patients manage pain at end-of-life. *PAIN®, 103*(1–2), 157–162.

Mills, N., Pajares, F., & Herron, C. (2007). Self-efficacy of college intermediate French students: Relation to achievement and motivation. *Language Learning, 57*(3), 417–442.

Murray, D. K., Sacheli, M. A., Eng, J. J., & Stoessl, A. J. (2014). The effects of exercise on cognition in Parkinson's disease: A systematic review. *Translational Neurodegeneration, 3*, 1–13.

Parkinson's Foundation. (2025a). *Cognitive changes*. Retrieved February 2025, from https://www.parkinson.org/understanding-parkinsons/non-movement-symptoms/cognitive

Parkinson's Foundation. (2025b). *Fatigue*. Retrieved February 2025, from https://www.parkinson.org/understanding-parkinsons/non-movement-symptoms/fatigue

Parkinson's Foundation. (2025c). *Pain in Parkinson's disease*. Retrieved February 2025, from https://www.parkinson.org/library/fact-sheets/pain

Rastgardani, T., Armstrong, M. J., Gagliardi, A. R., Grabovsky, A., & Marras, C. (2019). Communication about OFF periods in Parkinson's disease: A survey of physicians, patients, and carepartners. *Frontiers in Neurology, 10*, 892.

Saldert, C., & Bauer, M. (2017). Multifaceted communication problems in everyday conversations involving people with Parkinson's disease. *Brain Sciences*, 7(10), 123.

Schrag, A., Khan, K., Hotham, S., Merritt, R., Rascol, O., & Graham, L. (2018). Experience of care for Parkinson's disease in European countries: A survey by the European Parkinson's disease association. *European Journal of Neurology*, 25(12), 1410.e120.

Vassilev, I., Rogers, A., Kennedy, A., & Koetsenruijter, J. (2014). The influence of social networks on self-management support: A metasynthesis. *BMC Public Health*, 14(1), 1–12, Article 719. https://doi.org/10.1186/1471-2458-14-719

Vassilev, I., Rogers, A., Sanders, C., Kennedy, A., Blickem, C., Protheroe, J., Bower, P., Kirk, S., Chew-Graham, C., & Morris, R. (2011). Social networks, social capital and chronic illness self-management: A realist review. *Chronic Illness*, 7(1), 60–86.

Williams-Gray, C. H., Evans, J. R., Goris, A., Foltynie, T., Ban, M., Robbins, T. W., Brayne, C., Kolachana, B. S., Weinberger, D. R., Sawcer, S. J., & Barker, R. A. (2009). The distinct cognitive syndromes of Parkinson's disease: 5 year follow-up of the CamPaIGN cohort. *Brain*, 132(11), 2958–2969.

Williams-Gray, C. H., Foltynie, T., Brayne, C. E. G., Robbins, T. W., & Barker, R. A. (2007). Evolution of cognitive dysfunction in an incident Parkinson's disease cohort. *Brain*, 130(7), 1787–1798.

Wyatt, M. (2018). Language teachers' self-efficacy beliefs: An introduction. In S. Mercer & A. Kostoulas (Eds.), *Language teacher psychology*. Multilingual Matters.

Zaman, M. S., Ghahari, S., & McColl, M. A. (2021). Barriers to accessing healthcare services for people with Parkinson's disease: A scoping review. *Journal of Parkinson's Disease*, 11(4), 1537–1553.

4

WHAT LIFESTYLE CHANGES CAN I MAKE TO IMPROVE MY WELL-BEING?

Looking after your overall health becomes doubly important after a Parkinson's diagnosis. You want your body to be functioning at an optimal level to manage the challenges that Parkinson's brings, but also you do not want to introduce additional health issues. Basic principles like improving sleep, optimising nutrition, engaging in physical activity tailored to your needs, practising relaxation techniques, and taking your medication are all vital. We will look at them in turn here. These healthy behaviours are activities that can be directly or indirectly measured. Having the intention to eat three fruits a day is not a behaviour. Wanting to lose weight is a goal, but not a behaviour, but walking around the park every morning is a measurable activity linked to your intentions and goals.

It is complicated to determine what constitutes healthy behaviour and how much of it is actually needed. What is classified as healthy behaviour changes over time as medical knowledge advances and cultural and resource differences increase. In the 1950s, children were encouraged to eat the fat off meat, and in the USA in 1919, the dietary advice promoted a healthy meal of bread, milk, and cookies.

Your healthy behaviours are also somewhat independent; for example, you might be flossing your teeth every night and at the

DOI: 10.4324/9781003484332-5

same time have a lot of sugar in your diet. You might be exercising, but still drink to excess. Also, healthy behaviours are not stable over time. There might be a period in your life that going to work every day required you to walk at least 10,000 steps, but now that you are working from home you hardly have the chance to walk outside your apartment.

Also, these health behaviours and habits are motivated by our personal values, as we discussed in Chapter 2. Sometimes there might be a conflict in these values. We do value our health and want to go to sleep early to keep the body healthy and rested. At the same time, we also value spending time with loved ones and staying up late with your partner is also high on your values list. If while reading the following chapter you notice that conflicting values are an issue for you, choose one of the two or more values to focus on. That one value will guide you through the behaviour change process.

As we saw in earlier chapters, we tell ourselves stories of who we are, and we live by them. Because much of our self is formed pre-verbally, the beliefs that guide us can be hidden from us. We may have beliefs like 'I'm the sort of person who cannot control how much chocolate I eat, once I start, I don't stop' or 'I'm not sporty; I don't exercise'. If we get to know these stories we live by, we will be able to edit and change them if we need to. If we focus on such stories and see them from fresh angles, we can find new, more flexible ways of defining ourselves, others and everything around us. Your new story might be 'I'm the kind of person who needs to move every day to feel good'. These stories are powerful and can help with changing habits and behaviours.

It is best to focus on habits that are easy to start and track small wins. The brain thrives on dopamine boosts, even from tiny achievements. 'If-then' plans also help to create routines. These plans link cues with your behaviour. For example, 'If I pass the supermarket, I'll buy some salad to eat with my dinner'. This makes the habit easier to remember and execute. You can also use habit stacking, where you add new habits to existing routines. For example, you make coffee every morning when you wake up, and then you add a new habit straight after pouring your first cup of coffee, for example, taking your new medication.

4.1 HOW CAN I IMPROVE SLEEP WITH PARKINSON'S?

A good night's sleep is critical to our health and well-being. However, for people with Parkinson's, sleep becomes even more important as the body needs more time to restore and repair itself. The brain changes that are part of Parkinson's can also cause sleep difficulties, and some people have problems sleeping even before movement symptoms develop and Parkinson's is diagnosed. Some Parkinson's medications can disrupt sleep. Others make people sleepy during the day. Not surprisingly, sleep-related symptoms are reported by more than 75% of people with Parkinson's (Parkinson's Foundation, 2025).

Medication side effects might be responsible for these difficulties as well as difficulties to turn around in bed and get comfortable. Recurrent Parkinson's symptoms like disordered breathing, REM sleep behavioural disorder (i.e. when you physically act out vivid, often unpleasant dreams with vocal sounds and sudden, often violent arm and leg movements during REM sleep), restless leg syndrome and periodic limb movement can all contribute to difficulties getting to sleep and staying asleep. Disrupted sleep can affect your health, mood, and overall quality of life. Furthermore, when you don't sleep well, your care partner's sleep is disrupted, too. Care partners also need restful sleep to stay healthy and be at their best.

As I had discussed previously (Bogosian, 2020), a lot of people with a long-term health condition report not sleeping well or not feeling rested when they wake up, but this vague sense of restlessness can be narrowed to the specific issues with sleep. Several sleep experts reviewed more than 200 previously published sleep studies in an attempt to define more concretely what sort of sleep people should aspire to each night. They outlined the four criteria they landed on in a paper in *Sleep Health*, a journal run by the National

Sleep Foundation. Here, according to the report, are the criteria of a good night's sleep (Ohayon et al., 2017):

1. You take half an hour or less to fall asleep.
2. You wake up no more than once per night.
3. If you do wake up in the middle of the night, you fall back asleep within 20 minutes.
4. You are asleep for at least 85% of the time you spend in bed.

But how could you 'Get a good night's sleep'? The best you can do to improve on your sleep is to stop focusing on your lack of sleep. The brain is a problem-solving machine. When the problem is 'difficulty sleeping' the brain will get on overdrive trying to sort out this problem and all this brain activity will keep you awake all night. It is a bit like carrying a full cup of coffee on a tray, the more you look at the cup and not where you are going the more likely it is to spill the coffee. The more relaxed you are about it the more likely it is for the coffee to remain in the cup.

Thinking about sleep as something that sometimes doesn't happen, and it does not have huge effect in your life if it doesn't happen can be a more helpful approach to deal with the difficulty. Be compassionate and patient: it takes time and by being kind and relaxed around your sleep habits you remove unnecessary obstacles.

You can let go of worries about sleep and improve your sleep with simple sleep hygiene strategies.

First of all, let's move the focus away from the night sleep and on to how you spend the day. A day that is relatively busy and enjoyable with the right amount of relaxing breaks is more likely to have produce enough 'sleep drive' to lead to a good night's sleep. Whenever thoughts about how tired you feel or that you didn't have enough sleep or that you can't find energy to do anything, acknowledge the thoughts and let them go. Not sleeping well will make you less energetic the next day but most of the times the mind exacerbates the effects with focusing too much on this. OK, you did not have a great night, that was that, what can you do today to make the day fun.

A great way to enjoy your day is to plan it in advance. Having a plan the previous night, for example, three to five 'main' events will guide your day. The events could be something like going to the supermarket to pick up healthy snacks, walking your dog around the park, or sampling cakes at the newly open café in your neighbour-hood. Activities or events that get you moving and out of the house, experiencing things and interacting with other people.

Maya found her days really overwhelming as she was unable to do any simple task without a great amount of struggle and pain. So, she told me she always planned her day to do one 'big thing' a day. Something like taking her car to the garage or picking up her grandson from nursery and spending an hour with him until her daughter-in-law would come to pick him up. Her focus was the one task a day, and she would be delighted to tick it off. But she had some smaller tasks that she included in her daily list just for the thrill of ticking things off, the smaller tasks included things like taking the bins out or cleaning the cat's food bowl. No matter how you plan your day, make sure your overall week includes some tasks that make you feel effective and productive and give you a sense of achieve-ment and some enjoyable tasks, this way your days and weeks will feel happy and satisfying.

Parkinson's can vary from day to day, and unpredictability and uncertainty make planning difficult; you can use an altered version of daily planning. It might mean that you create a bucket list of things you would like to do or achieve, and depending on how you feel each day, you can pick up an item to do. Your list might include items that can be completed in a few minutes or others that will take most of the day. Take each day as it comes. The point is not to treat your bucket list as an infinite to-do list that will never get done, but as an ideas list, something to jog your memory of things you like to do, so you can bring more intention to your days.

Equally important is to build in some resting time during the day. Have an active, alive home with music, TV, chatter, and activity, indoors and outdoors, but built in resting times as well. It might be that a rhythm of an hour and a half productivity followed by a

15-minute break for 3 cycles, then followed by a 2-hour break, and another 2 cycles of an hour and a half activity and a 15-minute break will work for you, or a variation of such a rhythm. The timings are not important here, what is important is to build in your day a rhythm that will feel easy and natural to you. You could also have a mid-point reset into your day, where you take a short nap after lunch, and if not more than 1 hour, this nap can re-energise you for the second half of the day.

Prepare yourself and your environment to wind down the day and relax. Don't focus on the sleep itself, start wind things down. It is best to follow a similar routine every day, similar timings and similar activities, so both your mind and your body get into a pattern over time: for example, reading a book in low light, having a warm bath, having a cup of herbal tea, avoiding screens or socialising for an hour or two before you go to bed, avoiding strenuous physical activity before you go to bed – even though physical activity during the day can help you regulate your sleep and help you go to sleep easier at night – and doing something really vigorous just before bed will not be conducive to a good night's sleep. You may also want to ensure that the environment is relatively dark and peaceful.

A few years ago, I was discussing sleep difficulties with a group of people with Parkinson's, and people shared things that helped them feel comfortable, relaxed, and peaceful in the evenings before bed. Ian wore a pair of fresh pyjamas of breathable material. His issue was that he was getting sweaty in the night, and that woke him up, and then it was difficult to get back to sleep. So, a new pair of lighter, more breathable fabric pyjamas did the trick. Alexa and Louisa talked about melatonin tablets that you can purchase over the counter. Melatonin is a natural hormone that the brain produces in the late evening and throughout the night. Research shows that melatonin tablets help when taken several hours before bedtime. Alexa and Louisa also talked about using a 'light box', which is a lamp that turns slowly on and off when programmed. During the winter, especially when natural light is limited, our circadian rhythm can get disturbed, and so does our sleep. This artificial light mimicking daylight can help the body distinguish between day and night and adjust appropriately. Having regular massages was Pamela's tip to stay relaxed and sleep better. Massages can be expensive and feel too self-indulgent, but we are all allowed a few things on our 'luxuries' list, things that are somewhat expensive but make us feel happy and abundant, and Pamela was adamant that getting a massage was improving her quality of life and quality of sleep. Think about all the little things you spend money on that you don't really need or want, she said, you could spend it on something you like and enjoy. And it doesn't have to be too frequent, and you can find coupons and promotional deals to get massages for cheaper. Other practical tips were mentioned during the session, like avoiding drinking too much water before bed, avoiding caffeine and alcohol, and avoiding screens after 8 pm.

Having a few techniques that you know can help you relax is very useful, but relying too much on them can also have the opposite effect. In his brilliantly written and informative book, *The Sleep Book: How to Sleep Well Every Night,* Dr Guy Meadows urges his readers to adopt a balanced approach to sleep props. Don't get hooked on rigid sleep routines and rituals, he warns. Sleep is a natural and individualised thing. Take time, try different things to see what works for you. Usually, sleep happens when you stop the struggle.

Cognitive behavioural therapy has been empirically tested as a treatment for insomnia and found effective in reducing different sleep-related problems for people who experience sleep difficulties. In cognitive behavioural therapy, people are encouraged to identify, challenge, and replace dysfunctional beliefs and attitudes about sleep and insomnia. Such misconceptions may include unrealistic expectations of sleep, fear of missing out on sleep and overestimation of the consequences of poor sleep. Cognitive behavioural therapy also appears to be effective in treating depression and sleep disorders in people with Parkinson's, while psychoeducation programmes alone should be avoided (Zarotti et al., 2020).

Jon Kabat-Zinn, in his book, *Full Catastrophe Living: How to Cope with Stress, Pain and Illness Using Mindfulness Meditation*, talks about his insomnia. He describes how he stopped seeing insomnia as an issue and started seeing it as an opportunity to catch up on his writing or practice mindfulness meditation. Mindfulness meditation helps to acknowledge your thoughts and not let them bother you, to do what you want to do, regardless of what your thoughts have to say. In the night, you can use the touch of your duvet on your toes or the gentle movement of your chest as you breathe to ground yourself in the present moment and a place to return your attention when your mind wants to wander off. You can't stop your mind from having worrisome thoughts, but you can always choose how much you buy into them.

Another way to catch those thoughts that keep you awake is to write them down in a journal. Marcus Aurelius, the Roman Emperor from 161 to 180 AD, recorded his thoughts about what he learned from the day every night, reflected on the event, and wrote his ideas on what he saw and heard. These notes serve as a source of self-guidance and self-improvement. There is a lot to be said about the way we currently live our lives without a moment to really reflect on things and form our own opinions and writing down our thoughts can be a great way to process thoughts, feelings, and situations. It is also a way to recognise our thoughts and put them out of our mind and on paper. And if what you are writing happens to be about anxious thoughts it is important to move the notebook out of sight when you are done, as research shows that treating thoughts as material objects can increase or decrease their impact (Briñol et al., 2013), so if you write your thoughts and you keep the paper with you, it will act as a physical reminder and if you throw it away it will feel as if you have also discarded the thoughts it contains.

An easy trap that many of us fall into when we know that we mustn't think or stress about something is that we do, and then we stress even more in a vicious circle that can escalate indefinitely. Of course, you will worry about not sleeping and wonder how bad this will affect your day; there is no escaping that. The real challenge is can you be OK with having this worrisome thought? Don't indulge them; just look at them and nod as if saying to your thoughts: Cool, I see you've come again, but I don't have time to chat. I'd like to do something else.

To summarise, move your focus away from the worry that you are not sleeping well and direct your attention to simple habits that help with sleep. There is no point lying in bed unable to sleep for long periods of time, it is better to get up and do something else until you feel tired, then try to sleep again. Things like going to bed and getting up at around the same time every day, limiting caffeine and alcohol in the evenings, using the bed for sleep only, limiting daytime naps and increasing the things you do during the day will all help.

4.2 HOW CAN I OPTIMISE MY NUTRITION TO SUPPORT OVERALL HEALTH?

Nutrition is important for maintaining overall health, but it is especially important in Parkinson's. Compared to the general older population, a higher prevalence of malnutrition has been reported in Parkinson's. Depending on how 'malnutrition' was measured, the prevalence ranged from 0% to 24%, while 3–60% of people with Parkinson's were reported to be at risk of malnutrition (Sheard et al., 2011). Malnourishment can make us susceptible to infection and reduce our ability to exercise, which may contribute to poor quality of life. A decrease in muscle mass or lean body mass and abnormal fat distribution is also often observed in Parkinson's. The duration and the severity of Parkinson's have been linked to nutrition-related risk factors in Parkinson's (Fu et al., 2022).

Gastrointestinal symptoms, such as hyposmia, constipation, dysphagia, delayed gastric emptying, early satiety, and nausea, may reduce food intake and affect people's nutritional status. Dysphagia (difficulty eating) is believed to play a role in weight loss. However, according to some authors it makes a minor contribution, because it usually occurs in the advanced phases of the disease, although sometimes it is present at onset. Impaired gastric emptying is commonly reported in both early and advanced Parkinson's. It seems to be related to severe motor function impairment and motor fluctuations, typical of disease progression, but the basis of the association is not fully understood. Besides clinical symptoms, drug treatment may also affect your nutritional status. Dopamine replacement therapy is often used to treat motor symptoms, and the most commonly used medication is levodopa. Some of the most common side effects of levodopa are nausea, vomiting (affects food intake), and dyskinesia (increases energy expenditure). Moreover, large neutral amino acids in the diet compete with levodopa for absorption within the small intestine and transportation across the blood–brain barrier. Optimising drug treatment for both motor and non-motor symptoms is essential. Nutritional interventions and counselling that ensure nutritional balance can prevent weight loss or gain (Barichella et al., 2009).

Here we will talk about 'healthy eating'. 'Healthy eating' describes a variety of eating behaviours associated with good health and consistent with dietary guidelines, such as increased consumption of foods (or foods containing nutrients) conducive to good health, for example, fruits, vegetables, whole-grains, vitamins, and minerals; decreased consumption of foods (or nutrients) which when consumed in excess are associated with poor health, for example, fast food, sugar-sweetened beverages, saturated fat, sodium, sugar, and alcohol; decreased portion sizes of energy-dense foods; and adherence to diet patterns which align to good health.

A balanced diet rich in fruits, vegetables, whole grains, nuts and seeds, non-fried fish, olive oil, wine, coconut oil, fresh herbs, and spices and lean proteins can support overall health and may offer neuroprotective benefits in Parkinson's (Barichella et al., 2009; Mischley et al., 2017). These foods contribute to natural vitamins and polyphenols intake and reduce unsaturated fat ingestion. On the other hand, canned fruits and vegetables, diet and non-diet fizzy drinks, fried foods, beef, ice cream, yogurt, and cheese were associated with more rapid illness progression (Mischley et al., 2017).

Mediterranean diet involves all the above foods (fruits, vegetables, whole grains, lean proteins, and healthy fats) and is a diet that has been researched a lot in terms of effects it may have on Parkinson's. The effect of Mediterranean diet seems to be related to an overall equilibrium of macronutrients, polyphenols, and vitamins than a specific nutritional factor. Furthermore, the Mediterranean diet improves insulin activity in the gut microbiota, which is essential in maintaining healthy intestinal mucosa and reducing neuroinflammation in Parkinson's. A large number of studies showed that when following strictly the Mediterranean diet, it delayed the onset of Parkinson's and was significantly associated with slower progression, less motor symptoms, and increased cognitive function. Although we see a lot of those associations, the evidence is not robust enough to make certain claims.

As research continues to explore the effects of nutrition in Parkinson's, one area that's gained attention is the role of dietary supplements like omega-3 fatty acids, genistein (a soybean isoflavone), and vitamins like D, C, and E. While none of these are currently proven to slow the progression of Parkinson's, some have shown promise in animal studies or early human trials. Animal studies have also indicated that caffeine can be neuroprotective. Similarly, several reports have revealed that both black and green tea exert neuroprotective effects in Parkinson's animal models (Seidl et al., 2014).

As we age, our taste in food changes. Our tongue has fewer taste buds, and our sense of smell dulls. Parkinson's can also affect the ability to smell certain things (such as bananas, dill pickles, and liquorice), further impacting taste. The taste for sweets is the last to go, so the older you get, the more enjoyment you may get from eating sweet things. Drinking plenty of water will help keep your bones strong, boost energy, and help you with constipation. Try to incorporate small healthy eating habit in your day, eat a fruit or a crunchy vegetable when you feel peckish instead of cakes or crisps, have a glass of water next to you at all times, so you can sip throughout the day, aim to add a portion of vegetables at lunch and dinner. These physical improvements can help you feel more confident and in control of your body. Nutrition is not a substitute for medical care, but it is an important component to improved mood and overall sense of well-being.

4.3 WHAT ARE THE BENEFITS OF PHYSICAL ACTIVITY?

The role of exercise in the management of Parkinson's is well documented. Meta-analyses showed that people with Parkinson's who are more physically active have better global cognition, quality of life and less mental health challenges. Increased physical activity levels are also linked to better sleep quality and less chronic pain (Still et al., 2024). Research has also shown that exercise may have protective effects associated with the basal ganglia (known as neurogenesis) which results in improvement in dopamine transmission, increased brain blood flow and new formation of neuronal synapses which in turn can improve motor function (Petzinger et al., 2015), like bradykinesia and postural balance (Allen et al., 2011; Lauhoff et al., 2013; Ridgel et al., 2012). Neurogenesis can also result in a slowed progression of Parkinson's and improvements in motor control, particularly when exercise is carried out at vigorous intensities (Arcolin et al., 2015; Marxreiter et al., 2013). People sometimes report that exercise gives them a specific purpose for their lives and helps them become more confident in their own ability (Eriksson et al., 2013).

So, it does not come as a surprise to see evidence that exercise also improves mood. The effects of physical activity on non-motor symptoms in Parkinson's, particularly mental well-being data back to at least the 1980s but it has received more and more attention. This focus is in part motivated by the anti-depressant effects of physical exercise in people with mood disorders without Parkinson's. A study published at the *Journal of Affective Disorders*, that included 2,190 participants, on the effects of exercise on depressive symptoms, showed that higher rates of physical exercise was associated with lower ratings of depression but not anxiety (D'Angelantonio et al., 2022).

How does exercising the body helps combat depression? There are different ways that the body is linked with the mind. One is that exerting your body muscles causes some minor injuries. Your brain starts to produce endorphins to counteract the painful effects of this. And when you stop exercising the endorphin production drops, but not immediately. For a while – many minutes in some cases – those endorphins continue to be produced and continue to influence the brain. Many people report a feeling of great pleasure when this is happening. The endorphins don't merely dull the physical pain of exercise; they also dull the mental and emotional pain. Exercise also reduces inflammation via several different processes (inflammation, cytokines, toll-like receptors, adipose tissue and via the vagal tone), which can contribute to better health outcomes for those experiencing mood difficulties (Mikkelsen et al., 2017).

But what kind of exercise is most beneficial in Parkinson's? Interventions for people with Parkinson's focus of resistance training, balance, aerobic exercise, and flexibility conducted in an exercise or rehabilitative setting (Goodwin et al., 2008). These exercises can improve balance, walking speed, exercise tolerance, gait function, aerobic capacity, motor control, physical functioning, muscular strength, and flexibility in Parkinson's (Choi et al., 2020). Several studies emphasised the benefits of aerobic exercise to improve symptoms. Higher intensities of exercise seem more effective in suppressing symptoms than lower intensities (Schenkman et al., 2018).

Parkinson's impairs the ability to select appropriate motor commands and affects the internal cueing systems, making rhythmic motor tasks (e.g. walking) difficult (Krotinger & Loui, 2021). Dance, especially with rhythmic music, fosters brain activity related to movement (Sharp & Hewitt, 2014). Using music as a pleasurable rhythmical auditory cue can potentially bypass the impaired basal ganglia loop (Krotinger & Loui, 2021) and foster the natural synchronisation between auditory and motor systems (Heiberger et al., 2011). In this way, music-based movement can improve motor functions by promoting synchronisation of movement to the music, facilitating coordinated actions such as walking (Zhou et al., 2021). This strategy of internalising auditory cues for movement can be applied in daily activities, helping individuals synchronise their walking to mentally-generated musical rhythm (Holmes & Hackney, 2017).

Further, dance programs provide opportunities for social interactions, non-verbal communication, and self-improvement, re-establishing self-identity and a sense of usefulness (Bognar et al., 2017; Carroll et al., 2022). A 2024 review of 13 trials involving a total of 496 people with Parkinson's showed that dance had a positive impact on mental health and quality of life when compared to passive control groups, that is, groups that did not receive anything alternative. A more granular analysis of the data of the 13 trials showed that non-partnered dance and dance interventions with lower total dosages were particularly beneficial for mental health (Cheng et al., 2024). Dance also teaches safe movement transition strategies, which reduces the risk and fear of falling (Holmes & Hackney, 2017; Ventura et al., 2016). As a participant from the study of Holmes and Hackney (2017) expressed: 'what it really did for me was to say that I didn't have to be scared of every little thing' (p. 264). Dance also redirects your attention away from the symptoms and disease to focus consciously on movements (Earhart, 2009; Heiberger et al., 2011; Ventura et al., 2016).

Music accompaniment, in turn, may play a vital role in facilitating the release of neurotransmitters such as dopamine, serotonin, endorphins, and endocannabinoids (Kalyani et al., 2019; Rios Romenets et al., 2015; Zhou et al., 2021) that improve mood, reduce stress, and alleviate depressive and anxiety symptoms. A meta-analysis showed that music-based movement therapy significantly improved motor function, balance, freezing of gait, walking velocity, and mental health. However, no significant effects were observed on gait cadence, stride length, and quality of life (Zhou et al., 2021).

Despite the clear benefits of exercise and physical activity in Parkinson's, only 30% achieve recommended activity levels, some people are inactive for 70% of the day, and most people are less active than their age-matched peers. There are also different motivators for men and women to engage in physical activity. Women tend to be more motivated by enjoyment of the activity and social support whereas being male and married can indicate longer time spent performing exercise. Women with Parkinson's might not have enough time to devote to exercise and self-care due to the higher burden of work/family care.

Although people with Parkinson's experience increasing difficulties engaging in exercise as the disease progresses, previous research has indicated that personal factors, including believing exercise can help and believing you have the ability to exercise and not illness severity, will determine whether you will exercise or not. Receiving rewards for engaging in regular exercise and having a personal coach can also help continue home-based exercise programmes (Van der Kolk et al., 2019).

If you would like to increase your physical activity but you don't know how, try putting some of the things we learn in Chapter 2 in practice here, think of ways that physical activity links to your core values and how you want to show up in life to help you motivate yourself. Or you can rephrase your physical activity goal as a SMART goal, for example, I will walk with my partner on Wednesdays and Fridays, after dinner, around the park for 20 minutes. You could also think of two to three things that could get in the way of you achieving the goal and ways to overcome them. For example, fatigue in the evening can get in the way of you getting out for your walk, so you could say, if I feel fatigued and unable to go out after dinner with my husband, I'll go out in the following morning after breakfast, I'll walk to the supermarket and buy myself my favourite snack as a treat for having achieved my goal. You could also think of ways to increase your belief in you capabilities, think of similar goals you have achieved in the past, talking to other people with Parkinson's who have retain some physical activity or watching videos of people with Parkinson's talking about their experience with physical activity or demonstrating how they go about incorporating movement in their daily life. Sharing your goal to be more physical active with friends and family can also help by getting encouragement from those close to you. Increased knowledge around exercise, including the importance as well as certain techniques or available classes, could be useful (Tuijt et al., 2020). Care partners (Nunes et al., 2015), written plans or schedules (Hellqvist et al., 2018), and exercising in a group setting (Hellqvist et al., 2018) are important motivators that can support your physical activity goals.

Information on the importance of exercise is a key aspect. In an interview study we completed recently, people believed strongly in the benefits of exercise for Parkinson's, but experienced guilt about not exercising enough and frustration when symptoms made it harder to continue (Baron & Bogosian, 2024). They also reported increased mood and well-being, body image, competition, and camaraderie all contributed to motivate them to exercise. Having active partners, supportive work, and varied exercise options were among the important facilitators of long-term exercise.

Exercise is one of the most effective ways to manage Parkinson's symptoms, helping with everything from balance and strength to mood and motivation. Engaging in any level of physical activity is beneficial for movement symptoms. If you are experiencing mild to moderate Parkinson's, targeted exercises can address specific symptoms. For example, aerobic exercise can improve fitness, walking exercises assist in gait, and resistance training strengthens muscles. Tango and other forms of dancing can also help improve motor symptoms, balance, and walking speed. Exercise may also improve cognition, depression, and fatigue.

4.4 HOW DO I MANAGE STRESS?

Your feelings are valid and allowed and they are not a waste of time. Feeling stressed does not mean that you're doing the wrong thing. You do not need to be perfect. You do not need to be positive and happy all the time. This section is for when you've been in that rut, when you feel stress has an effect on your mental health and mobility (Goltz et al., 2024), and you are ready to take the steps to feel reassured, feel relieved, and feel motivated to take your life back on again.

Avoiding stress is a battle that you can never win. It is impossible to control your environment. Stress can come from any direction when you least expect it. There will be rude people, broken computers, mixed-up dates of medical appointments, traffic, and broken water pipes. Also, there is the 'positive stress' that you don't want to miss out on, the stress that accompanies happy and essential changes, such as meeting new people, going to social functions, taking up new hobbies, initiating difficult but necessary discussions with loved ones. We cannot control the stressors, but we can mostly control our response to those stressors.

There is a four-step process to help you identify stressors and find ways to best deal with them.

Step 1: Write down your current stressors. Some of them are illness-related, such as pain or fatigue, dealing with a range of healthcare staff, hospital environment, and treatments. Others are emotional or social, such as preserving emotional balance, self-image and sense of mastery and control, sustaining existing relationships, and managing uncertainty.

Step 2: Score each stressor on a scale 1 to 5 on how much control you feel you have over them. For example, you might feel more in control when you are moving to a new house because there are tangible things you can do to address this stressor. You can ask people for advice on different locations, you can sign up with a few estate agencies to send you information about houses that are available to rent, and you can ask an occupational therapist about home modifications. You can score this stressor as may be a 4 out of 10. On the other hand, the uncertainty of the prognosis of your condition is stressful, but not much can be done. You can read about it on relevant and reliable websites, you can ask your doctor for more information so that you know what the likely progression or treatments scenarios are, but you won't be able to tell for sure how your condition will develop. So, you might score this stressor as a 2 out of 10.

Step 3: Once you have identified the challenges and how much control you have over them, you can start thinking about the strategies to manage those challenges. 'Emotion-focused' strategies are more helpful for demands we don't have much power over. These help you manage your emotions around the challenge. Such strategies might include writing a diary about what is happening and how you feel about things, talking to friends about what worries you, taking a yoga or meditation class to help with acceptance or even taking up a creative hobby to help you express your emotions through art.

Mind-body exercises like mindfulness, Tai Chi, Qigong, and yoga have become increasingly popular for people with Parkinson's. In fact, 32% of 5,000 people surveyed indicated to use relaxation exercises like Tai Chi or yoga at least several times per month to reduce stress. Tai Chi and Qigong both describe traditional Chinese martial art forms of training, which include breathing and meditation exercises alongside controlled body movements. Randomised control trials investigating the effects of Qigong and Tai Chi with regards to stress-related symptoms are limited, but overall show promising results in improving quality of life and mood. Yoga, a Hindu relaxation technique involving specific body postures and breathing exercises, has also been studied in a recent meta-analysis. We have positive, albeit limited, empirical evidence around the effects of yoga in Parkinson's with regard to functional mobility, balance, and quality of life (Suarez-Iglesias et al., 2022). You can search for yoga classes that focus on long-term conditions or generic ones. If you live in a big city, it is very likely there will be meditation centres that you can join but also the internet is full of free meditation practices that you can try. Mindfulness-based interventions encourage individuals to independently self-manage and adapt to the challenges created by their condition. In Parkinson's, emerging clinical evidence suggests that mindfulness-based interventions may reduce psychological distress and improve clinical symptoms (Bogosian et al., 2022; van der Heide et al., 2021). Furthermore, alternative treatment methods like sensory focused exercise, acupuncture, bright light therapy, or singing have been suggested for stress-alleviation in Parkinson's.

For the stressors that you do have more control over, 'problem-focused' strategies might be the best way forward; taking baby steps to resolve the issue actively. Take cognitive difficulties, for example, which manifests as difficulty concentrating, paying attention and working through problems. Often it prevents you from completing work tasks on time and to the standards you want them. To solve this issue, you can ask your employer to give you the most important tasks early on in the day, and not surprise you with new demands at 3 pm. You can delegate some of the tasks that are not the core of your job to other colleagues. This will not only reduce your workload, but also teach you a valuable skill: appropriately delegating tasks to the right people, giving them specific instructions, and following up on progress. Another thing you can do is to say 'no' to jobs that are not relevant to what you have been employed to do. In other words, cut down any 'volunteer work' you do for your employer and stick to the tasks that are required of you.

Another way that can help you feel in control is to approach stressful situations differently. When presented with a problem, stretch your imagination to find new and innovative solutions. Before giving up or opting for half-measures, try to think of alternatives. As with every skill the more you practice the better you become at it; you can also get more ideas if you talk to others or observe them to see how they find solutions to issues. Finally, another way to sharpen your problem-solving skills is to learn more about your problem, or your condition. More information usually gives us more ideas.

Planning and managing your time efficiently can also reduce unnecessary stress. For example, having to buy a present for someone if left for the last minute can be a stressful experience but it can be a pleasant activity if we are out in the shops early enough to give us time to browse and choose wisely. Use any tools that appeal to you. Notebooks, post-it notes, Excel spreadsheets, mobile phone apps, anything that can help you plan what needs to be done and when, and to help you remember the plans you made. Being prepared can save you from a lot of unnecessary stress.

Another way to reduce stress or handle it better is to discuss your intention to manage stress better openly and respectfully. Express your needs and ask for what you want. Try to avoid the trap of accusations and opt to start with 'I' statements followed by the way you feel followed by the reason you feel this way. 'I feel ignored when you look at your phone when we're having dinner' rather than 'You always ignore me'. This invites open communication. People are less likely to get defensive or argue with how you feel. You feel how you feel, and you model a way for them also to express their feelings.

Other people can be a great source of comfort, and different people can help in various ways that are all equally valuable. Having someone understand what you are going through and offer love and trust is invaluable and can help you see the situation from different perspectives. People can also provide tangible support and help you sort out issues that cause you stress. Friends, family, and acquaintances can also help by giving advice, suggestions and information. They can make you aware of things you wouldn't have even thought to ask or to search for yourself. Finally, others can also give you feedback in certain situations and review with you what went wrong and how to fix things. Read also Chapter 5 for ideas to improve your communication and deepen your relationships.

Combining these techniques can yield the best results. Let's say you are stressing about a forthcoming airplane journey, lying awake at night wondering what you are going to do if you need the loo on the plane or how you would cope with the fatigue you are bound to feel in a 12-hour flight, etc. Try to replace any unhelpful thoughts with more helpful; 'There is no way I can travel on a plane for so long on my own' could become a less threatening one like 'It may be challenging, but a lot of people in my circumstances have done it, and it was OK'. With planning and forethought, you could prepare well ahead of the journey by searching online for travel tips and contacting specialised travel agencies. Finally, you could reduce your feelings of anxiety by regularly practising deep breathing.

Step 4: Finally, write down your metric of success. How will you know that you have addressed the problem sufficiently? A measure of success might be that your to-do list is no longer than five items each day, or that you no longer feel completely wiped out at the end of the day.

It is important to be flexible with your stress management techniques. We all have our favourite go-to strategies. Parkinson's will require you to consider new strategies as the condition or life circumstances change. That is why it is helpful from time to time to review the ways you've chosen to manage stress.

4.5 HOW TO REMEMBER TO TAKE THE MEDICATIONS?

For many people living with Parkinson's, taking medication isn't as simple as just popping a pill. It is a daily juggling act. Most people take several different medications throughout the day, and as Parkinson's changes over time, so do their prescriptions. What worked last year or even last week might suddenly stop being effective.

It is no surprise, then, that medication often shapes the entire rhythm of a person's day. Many people reported organising everything, meals, outings, exercise, appointments, around when their medication worked best. This helped them stay more comfortable and avoid symptom flare-ups in public. But it can also make life feel rigid, sometimes interfering with spontaneity or making simple plans more complicated than they should be. That's why medication management often becomes a team effort, with care partners playing a vital role in organising, tracking, and reminding.

But even with support, managing medication can be frustrating. Parkinson's symptoms can be unpredictable, and medication effectiveness may vary from one day to the next. Many people described using trial and error to figure out what helps most is tweaking doses, changing the timing of medications, or paying close attention to how sleep, food, and exercise affect how they feel.

One common challenge is the 'wearing-off' effect. This happens when medication stops working before the next dose is due, causing symptoms like tremor or stiffness to return. It can be alarming when the return of visible symptoms makes people feel like their medication has failed or draws unwanted attention. Adjusting the timing or dosage can help, but that process takes time, patience, and often, guidance from a healthcare provider. Some people also report that they are not always sure their medication was helping, especially when they didn't feel different, even though their loved ones noticed improvement.

Many people receiving regular medication who have not experienced adverse effects are still worried about possible problems in the future. These often arise from the belief that regular use can lead to dependence, or that the medication will accumulate within the body and lead to long-term effects. These issues are the social representations of medicine as being harmful and over-used. Side effects add another layer of complexity. These can range from dry mouth and drowsiness to more serious issues like hallucinations, insomnia, impulsive behaviour, or disturbing dreams. For some, the side effects are so difficult that they feel forced to choose between less control over their symptoms or living with uncomfortable side effects. For others, who experience depression, remembering to take their medication and taking the right doses becomes harder (Radojević et al., 2022).

Try to discuss some of these concerns with your healthcare team. For example, it might be worth learning about the active ingredients of the drug. How and when it is best to take them? What are the potential side effects? In which cases do you need to alert your doctor, for example, when specific side effects appear. How does the medication benefit your condition. When to expect to see benefits or what will happen with your condition if you don't take the medication. Your healthcare provider will welcome your interest and see this as an opportunity to work with you more collaboratively. You have a common goal of finding the best type of treatment regime, one that is the most convenient for you with the fewest side effects.

Across studies, researchers found that medication management was a key part of how people handled Parkinson's. Some used alarms, pill organisers, or relied on caregivers for reminders. People emphasised the importance of being included in decisions about their treatment, feeling informed, heard, and respected. Clear communication with healthcare professionals made a big difference in reducing confusion, improving trust, and helping people understand how medication plans were tailored to their unique symptoms and needs. It is useful to discuss with your healthcare provider your concerns about potential adverse effects of the medication and any doubts about the necessity of the medication. They might be able to provide you with new information to consider before making any choices about your healthcare plan.

Forgetfulness, complex schedules, and everyday distractions also make it hard to keep up with medications, particularly when work or social events get in the way. Timing matters a lot with Parkinson's medication. Some drugs must be taken with food, others on an empty stomach, and certain foods may interfere with how medications work. A quick and easy way to remember to take your medication at the right time is by using prompts. These prompts can be post-it notes at high visibility areas in the house (above the kettle?). Or you might want to bundle medicine taking with a well-established routine that happens at the intervals you need to take your medication. For example, you need to take your medicine once a day. You always without fail have to eat breakfast each morning, so what about merging taking your medication with having breakfast? Finding a system to monitor the dosage or whether you took the medication that day is also essential. For example, you might want to buy the seven-day pillboxes so you have a visual reminder and monitoring device at once. Or you can simply place a tick on the wall calendar once you take your medication. To help you remember to take your medications as you have planned it might help to associate taking your medication with a specific time (time-based retrieval). For example, it is 3 pm., meaning it is the time that you always take your medication. Also, you can associate taking your medication with a specific event (event-based retrieval). For example, finishing your dinner means you take your medication.

The most common and the most manageable issue to address is lack of understanding of the instructions, of what needs to be done. How often does the medication need to be taken, will you be able to open the bottle, know how to inject? If something is not 100% clear to you, ask for clarification. Doctors and nurses are happy to explain, and you will be helping future patients as doctors and nurses will become aware of the lack of clarity. Researchers have found that one of the most effective ways to improve adherence to medication is the 'teach-back' method. When a health professional is explaining to you what, how, when, and what ifs of taking medications, you then explain back what you have understood from their explanations.

Taking medication for Parkinson's can be complicated, frustrating, and at times unpredictable. Some days the medication works well, while on others, symptoms return sooner than expected. This 'wearing-off' effect when meds lose their impact before the next dose can be unsettling. What helps? Knowledge and communication. Understanding how your medication works, how and when to take it, and what side effects to look out for can empower you to take control. Talk to your doctor and ask questions, voice concerns, and work together to find the best plan for *you*. Being included in these decisions makes a huge difference. Setting up systems to remind you to take the medication can also help. With the right support and strategies, it becomes easier to stay on track and feel more in control of your health.

FURTHER READING

Some helpful books and other resources on lifestyle changes.

British Psychological Society. (2021). *Supporting people with neurodegenerative conditions* Retrieved June 4, 2025, from https://www.bps.org.uk/news/new-guidance-supporting-people-neurodegenerative-conditions

Kabat-Zinn, J. (2023). *Wherever you go, there you are: Mindfulness meditation in everyday life*. Hachette UK.

Meadows, G. (2014). *The sleep book: How to sleep well every night*. Hachette UK.

Parkinson's Foundation. (n.d.). *Diet and nutrition*. Retrieved June 4, 2025, from https://www.parkinson.org/living-with-parkinsons/management/diet-nutrition

Parkinson's UK. (n.d.). *Information and support on physical activity and exercise*. Retrieved June 4, 2025, from https://www.parkinsons.org.uk/information-and-support/physical-activity-and-exercise

Parkinson's UK. (n.d.). *Staying active at home with Parkinson's: Your toolkit*. Retrieved June 4, 2025, from https://www.parkinsons.org.uk/information-and-support/staying-active-home-parkinsons-your-toolkit

REFERENCES

Allen, N. E., Sherrington, C., Paul, S. S., & Canning, C. G. (2011). Balance and falls in Parkinson's disease: A meta-analysis of the effect of exercise and motor training. *Movement Disorders*, *26*(9), 1605–1615.

Arcolin, I., Pisano, F., Delconte, C., Godi, M., Schieppati, M., Mezzani, A., Picco, D., Grasso, M., & Nardone, A. (2015). Intensive cycle ergometer training improves gait speed and endurance in patients with Parkinson's disease: A comparison with treadmill training. *Restorative Neurology and Neuroscience*, *34*(1), 125–138.

Barichella, M., Cereda, E., & Pezzoli, G. (2009). Major nutritional issues in the management of Parkinson's disease. *Movement Disorders*, *24*(13), 1881–1892.

Baron, F., & Bogosian, A. (2024). Exploring social, cultural and environmental factors that influence attitudes to exercise among people with Parkinson's disease: A qualitative study. *Journal of Health Psychology*, 13591053241296647.

Bognar, S., DeFaria, A. M., O'Dwyer, C., Pankiw, E., Simic Bogler, J., Teixeira, S., Nyhof-Young, J., & Evans, C. (2017). More than just dancing: Experiences of people with Parkinson's disease in a therapeutic dance program. *Disability and Rehabilitation*, *39*(11), 1073–1078. https://doi.org/10.1080/09638288.2016.1175037

Bogosian, A. (2020). *Living well with a long-term health condition: An evidence-based guide to managing your symptoms*. Routledge.

Bogosian, A., Hurt, C. S., Hindle, J. V., McCracken, L. M., Vasconcelos e Sa, D. A., Axell, S., Tapper, K., Stevens, J., Hirani, P. S., Salhab, M., Ye, W., & Cubi-Molla, P. (2022). Acceptability and feasibility of a mindfulness intervention delivered via videoconferencing for people with Parkinson's. *Journal of Geriatric Psychiatry and Neurology*, *35*(1), 155–167.

Briñol, P., Gascó, M., Petty, R. E., & Horcajo, J. (2013). Treating thoughts as material objects can increase or decrease their impact on evaluation. *Psychological science*, *24*(1), 41–47.

Carroll, S. J., Dale, M. J., & Bail, K. (2022). Out and proud . . . in all your shaking glory' the wellbeing impact of a dance program with public dance performance for people with Parkinson's disease: A qualitative study. *Disability and Rehabilitation*, *45*(20), 1–12. https://doi.org/10.1080/096382 88.2022.2122598

Cheng, W. H., Quan, Y., & Thompson, W. F. (2024). The effect of dance on mental health and quality of life of people with Parkinson's disease: A systematic review and three-level meta-analysis. *Archives of Gerontology and Geriatrics*, *120*, 105326.

Choi, H. Y., Cho, K. H., Jin, C., Lee, J., Kim, T. H., Jung, W. S., Moon, S. K., Ko, C. N., Cho, S. Y., Jeon, C. Y., Choi, T. Y., Lee, M. S., Lee, S.-H., Chung, E. K., & Kwon, S. (2020). Exercise therapies for Parkinson's disease: A systematic review and meta-analysis. *Parkinson's Disease*, *2020*(1), 2565320.

D'Angelantonio, M., Collins, J. L., Manchia, M., Baldessarini, R. J., & Tondo, L. (2022). Physical exercise, depression, and anxiety in 2190 affective disorder subjects. *Journal of Affective Disorders*, *309*, 172–177.

Earhart, G. M. (2009). Dance as therapy for individuals with Parkinson's disease. *European Journal of Physical and Rehabilitation Medicine*, *45*(2), 231–238.

Eriksson, B. M., Arne, M., & Ahlgren, C. (2013). Keep moving to retain the healthy self: The meaning of physical exercise in individuals with Parkinson's disease. *Disability and Rehabilitation*, *35*(26), 2237–2244.

Fu, J., Li, Z., Wang, F., & Yu, K. (2022). Prevalence of malnutrition/malnutrition risk and nutrition-related risk factors among patients with Parkinson's disease: Systematic review and meta-analysis. *Nutritional Neuroscience*, *25*, 2228–2238.

Goltz, F., van der Heide, A., & Helmich, R. C. (2024). Alleviating stress in Parkinson's disease: Symptomatic treatment, disease modification, or both? *Journal of Parkinson's Disease*, *14*(s1), S147–S158.

Goodwin, V. A., Richards, S. H., Taylor, R. S., Taylor, A. H., & Campbell, J. L. (2008). The effectiveness of exercise interventions for people with Parkinson's disease: A systematic review and meta-analysis. *Movement Disorders*, *23*(5), 631–640.

Heiberger, L., Maurer, C., Amtage, F., Mendez-Balbuena, I., Schulte-Mönting, J., Hepp-Reymond, M. C., & Kristeva, R. (2011). Impact of a weekly dance class on the functional mobility and on the quality of life of individuals with Parkinson's disease. *Frontiers in Aging Neuroscience*, *3*, 14.

Hellqvist, C., Dizdar, N., Hagell, P., Berterö, C., & Sund-Levander, M. (2018). Improving self-management for persons with Parkinson's disease through education focusing on management of daily life: Patients' and relatives' experience of the Swedish National Parkinson School. *Journal of Clinical Nursing, 27*(19–20), 3719–3728.

Holmes, W. M., & Hackney, M. E. (2017). Adapted tango for adults with Parkinson's disease: A qualitative study. *Adapted Physical Activity Quarterly, 34*(3), 256–275. https://doi.org/10.1123/apaq.2015-0113

Kalyani, H. H. N., Sullivan, K. A., Moyle, G., Brauer, S., Jeffrey, E. R., & Kerr, G. K. (2019). Impacts of dance on cognition, psychological symptoms and quality of life in Parkinson's disease. *NeuroRehabilitation (Reading, Mass.), 45*(2), 273–283. https://doi.org/10.3233/NRE-192788

Krotinger, A., & Loui, P. (2021). Rhythm and groove as cognitive mechanisms of dance intervention in Parkinson's disease. *PLOS One, 16*(5), Article e0249933. https://doi.org/10.1371/journal.pone.0249933

Lauhoff, P., Murphy, N., Doherty, C., & Horgan, N. F. (2013). A controlled clinical trial investigating the effects of cycle ergometry training on exercise tolerance, balance and quality of life in patients with Parkinson's disease. *Disability and Rehabilitation, 35*(5), 382–387.

Marxreiter, F., Regensburger, M., & Winkler, J. (2013). Adult neurogenesis in Parkinson's disease. *Cellular and Molecular Life Sciences, 70*, 459–473.

Mikkelsen, K., Stojanovska, L., Polenaković, M., Bosevski, M., & Apostolopoulos, V. (2017). Exercise and mental health. *Maturitas.* https://doi.org/10.1016/j.maturitas.2017.09.003

Mischley, L. K., Lau, R. C., & Bennett, R. D. (2017). Role of diet and nutritional supplements in Parkinson's disease progression. *Oxidative Medicine and Cellular Longevity, 2017*(1), 6405278.

Nunes, F., & Fitzpatrick, G. (2015). Self-care technologies and collaboration. *International Journal of Human-Computer Interaction, 31*(12), 869–881.

Ohayon, M., Wickwire, E. M., Hirshkowitz, M., Albert, S. M., Avidan, A., Daly, F. J., Dauvilliers, Y., Ferri, R., Fung, C., Gozal, D., & Hazen, N. (2017). National Sleep Foundation's sleep quality recommendations: First report. *Sleep Health, 3*(1), 6–19.

Parkinson's Foundation. (2025). *Sleep disorders.* Retrieved May 2025, from https://www.parkinson.org/understanding-parkinsons/non-movement-symptoms/sleep-disorders

Petzinger, G. M., Holschneider, D. P., Fisher, B. E., McEwen, S., Kintz, N., Halliday, M., Toy, W., Walsh, J. W., Beeler, J., & Jakowec, M. W. (2015). The effects of exercise on dopamine neurotransmission in Parkinson's disease: Targeting neuroplasticity to modulate basal ganglia circuitry. *Brain Plasticity*, *1*(1), 29–39.

Radojević, B., Dragašević-Mišković, N. T., Milovanović, A., Svetel, M., Petrović, I., Pešić, M., Tomić, A., Stanisavljević, D., Savić, M. M., & Kostić, V. S. (2022). Adherence to medication among Parkinson's disease patients using the adherence to refills and medications scale. *International Journal of Clinical Practice*, *2022*(1), 6741280.

Ridgel, A. L., Peacock, C. A., Fickes, E. J., & Kim, C. H. (2012). Active-assisted cycling improves tremor and bradykinesia in Parkinson's disease. *Archives of Physical Medicine and Rehabilitation*, *93*(11), 2049–2054.

Rios Romenets, S., Anang, J., Fereshtehnejad, S.-M., Pelletier, A., & Postuma, R. (2015). Tango for treatment of motor and non-motor manifestations in Parkinson's disease: A randomized control study. *Complementary Therapies in Medicine*, *23*(2), 175–184. https://doi.org/10.1016/j.ctim.2015.01.015

Schenkman, M., Moore, C. G., Kohrt, W. M., Hall, D. A., Delitto, A., Comella, C. L., Josbeno, D. A., Christiansen, C. L., Berman, B. D., Kluger, B. M., Melanson, E. L., Jain, S., Robichaud, J. A., Poon, C., & Corcos, D. M. (2018). Effect of high-intensity treadmill exercise on motor symptoms in patients with de novo Parkinson disease: A phase 2 randomized clinical trial. *JAMA Neurology*, *75*(2), 219–226.

Seidl, S. E., Santiago, J. A., Bilyk, H., & Potashkin, J. A. (2014). The emerging role of nutrition in Parkinson's disease. *Frontiers in Aging Neuroscience*, *6*, 74578.

Sharp, K., & Hewitt, J. (2014). Dance as an intervention for people with Parkinson's disease: A systematic review and meta-analysis. *Neuroscience and Biobehavioral Reviews*, *47*, 445–456. https://doi.org/10.1016/j.neubiorev.2014.09.009

Sheard, J. M., Ash, S., Silburn, P. A., & Kerr, G. K. (2011). Prevalence of malnutrition in Parkinson's disease: A systematic review. *Nutrition Reviews*, *69*(9), 520–532.

Still, A., Hale, L., Alam, S., Morris, M. E., & Jayakaran, P. (2024). Relationships between physical activities performed under free-living conditions and non-motor symptoms in people with Parkinson's: A systematic review and meta-analysis. *Clinical Rehabilitation*. https://doi.org/10.1177/02692155241272967

Suarez-Iglesias, D., Santos, L., Sanchez-Lastra, M. A., & Ayan, C. (2022). Systematic review and meta-analysis of randomised controlled trials on the effects of yoga in people with Parkinson's disease. *Disability and Rehabilitation*, *44*(21), 6210–6229.

Tuijt, R., Tan, A., Armstrong, M., Pigott, J., Read, J., Davies, N., Walters, K., & Schrag, A. (2020). Self-management components as experienced by people with Parkinson's disease and their carers: A systematic review and synthesis of the qualitative literature. *Parkinson's Disease*, *2020*(1), 8857385.

van der Heide, A., Meinders, M. J., Speckens, A. E., Peerbolte, T. F., Bloem, B. R., & Helmich, R. C. (2021). Stress and mindfulness in Parkinson's disease: Clinical effects and potential underlying mechanisms. *Movement Disorders*, *36*(1), 64–70.

Van der Kolk, N. M., de Vries, N. M., Kessels, R. P., Joosten, H., Zwinderman, A. H., Post, B., & Bloem, B. R. (2019). Effectiveness of home-based and remotely supervised aerobic exercise in Parkinson's disease: A double-blind, randomised controlled trial. *The Lancet Neurology*, *18*(11), 998–1008.

Ventura, M. I., Barnes, D. E., Ross, J. M., Lanni, K. E., Sigvardt, K. A., & Disbrow, E. A. (2016). A pilot study to evaluate multi-dimensional effects of dance for people with Parkinson's disease. *Contemporary Clinical Trials*, *51*, 50–55. https://doi.org/10.1016/j.cct.2016.10.001

Zarotti, N., Eccles, F., Foley, J. A., Paget, A., Gunn, S., Leroi, I., & Simpson, J. (2020). Psychological interventions for people with Parkinson's disease in the early 2020s: Where do we stand? *Psychology and Psychotherapy: Theory, Research and Practice*. https://doi.org/10.1111/papt.12321

Zhou, Z., Zhou, R., Wei, W., Luan, R., & Li, K. (2021). Effects of music-based movement therapy on motor function, balance, gait, mental health, and quality of life for patients with Parkinson's disease: A systematic review and meta-analysis. *Clinical Rehabilitation*, *35*(7), 937–951. https://doi.org/10.1177/0269215521990526

5

HOW DOES PARKINSON'S AFFECT FAMILY RELATIONSHIPS AND FRIENDSHIPS?

Living with Parkinson's can affect how you connect with others. Many people with Parkinson's find that social situations become more difficult over time or that the diagnosis and its progression have reshaped the dynamics within their closest relationships. You may worry about how others see you, feel embarrassed about symptoms like facial masking or speech changes, or simply feel too tired to engage. These feelings are completely valid and very common.

Parenting and family roles also adapt in response to the shifting terrain of the disease. For individuals no longer able to work, family life sometimes takes on a renewed centrality, with parenting becoming a more prominent source of identity and purpose (Perepezko et al., 2019). Importantly, one early study found no difference in parental satisfaction between people with Parkinson's and age-matched peers, suggesting that core family roles may remain resilient despite illness challenges (Singer, 1974).

Outside of the family unit, social connections play a crucial role in maintaining quality of life, but these, too, can shift after diagnosis. Although many people report that their number of friends remains stable over time, studies show people with Parkinson's may become

DOI: 10.4324/9781003484332-6

less likely to initiate social outings or feel confident navigating public settings (Soleimani et al., 2016).

One of the hardest parts of Parkinson's can be how it makes you feel about being around other people. For some, staying home becomes easier than explaining symptoms or risking being misunderstood. Over time, this can lead to social withdrawal, spending less time with friends and family, or avoiding new connections. Loneliness is when you have people around you, but feel alone or disconnected. Loneliness can have a real impact on your mental and physical health as well as the medical care people receive. Connecting even to a few close people can make a huge difference. Research shows that having a strong support system and meaningful relationships can help protect your health, improve your mood, and even help your brain stay sharper.

Loneliness can also affect care partners. Care partners often report high levels of stress, fatigue, and loneliness, especially when their social life starts being impacted. Also, care partners with low self-efficacy (confidence in their abilities to manage the challenges) might be more vulnerable. Being aware of this can help you and your partner be more proactive in building support around both of you even when it is not needed, but it would be there if and when it is needed. Making sure both you and your partner have one social interaction a day is a good start and it can be something you do together or individually.

5.1 HOW DOES PARKINSON'S AFFECT INTIMACY, AND HOW CAN I IMPROVE EMOTIONAL CONNECTION WITH MY PARTNER?

After your Parkinson's diagnosis, your relationship with your partner might change. That doesn't mean something is wrong with you or your relationship; it just means you're learning how to adapt together. Some people have reported feeling closer to their partners, while others felt further apart. Let's look at what influences these changes and what you can do to stay connected and supported through the changes.

Not only the diagnosis but also different Parkinson's-related treatments can impact the couple's relationship. Deep brain stimulation was found in some cases to diminish sexual desire and, in some cases, worsen marital satisfaction (Perepezko et al., 2019). Whereas sexual desire seems to be lower after surgery, sexual satisfaction and the number of monthly initiations of sexual intercourse seemed not to change after surgery for people with advanced Parkinson's (Boel et al., 2016). In another study, 17 out of 24 couples reported experiencing marital conflict after subthalamic nucleus (SNT) stimulation (Schupbach et al., 2006). Agid et al. (2006) explained this worsened marital quality following surgery: either people living with Parkinson's rejected their spouse after they felt 'cured', or they were rejected by their spouse, who expected them to be able to return to how things were before the diagnosis following surgery.

Shifting relational roles (with more responsibility falling on the care partner), changes in sexual intimacy, engaging in fewer activities together, and financial burden (Perepezko et al., 2019) all contribute to strain in personal relationships. Researchers have also found that symptoms like reduced facial expression (called 'facial masking') and more advanced severity of the symptoms can also affect a couple's relationship (Gunnery et al., 2016). Finally, mood disorders and social difficulties, like depression, anxiety, negative social exchanges, and alexithymia (i.e. difficulty in experiencing, identifying, and expressing emotions), were associated with reduced relationship satisfaction (Perepezko et al., 2019). On the other hand, older couples and those who could better cope with the disease report better relationships. Spouses who report 'benefit finding', or ability to experience positive change when faced with a stressor like Parkinson's (Mavandadi et al., 2014), and affirmations of their commitment to each other after the diagnosis (Perepezko et al., 2019) also report higher relationship satisfaction.

A consistent theme across the literature is the importance of early and open communication about the disease. For example, having someone with you when you're attending a medical appointment for diagnosis results could be beneficial (Fleming et al., 2004), or sharing information about Parkinson's with other people can help them understand your situation (Kang & Ellis-Hill, 2015). However, this openness is not always effortless. Some individuals reported hesitating to disclose the full extent of their challenges to shield their children or protect family members from worry. This desire to maintain a sense of normalcy or avoid being a burden can lead to emotional distancing (Fleming et al., 2004).

Sexual desire and satisfaction can change, too. This is especially true for those who were diagnosed at a younger age and have more severe motor symptoms, fatigue, and rigidity. Researchers also reported that sex life satisfaction was significantly associated with marital satisfaction (Perepezko et al., 2019). Women also described changes in sexual relationships along with changes in body image and increased dependence on their partners, all affecting their relationships and increasing their sense of isolation (Fleming et al., 2004). People living with Parkinson's, especially women, believe the nonsexual aspects of their relationship became more important after the Parkinson's diagnosis (Buhmann et al., 2017).

You could show intimacy in many different non-sexual ways during the day to build up your connection, while you navigate the changes that Parkinson's has brought you. It could be a hug when your partner is doing the dishes, holding hands while watching your favourite show, leaning on their shoulder when working on a crossword puzzle. In an earlier chapter, we saw the many benefits of physical exercise, including dancing. These benefits extend to relationships as well. For example, attending tango sessions can improve functioning within family roles (Zafar et al., 2017). These small touches during the day will help to start building a new language of expressing affection, your love, and appreciation for your partner, and teach you ways to stay connected. Being creative and flexible in finding ways to connect emotionally can help maintain a sense of closeness and intimacy despite the challenges posed by Parkinson's.

After Parkinson's, relationships can shift. One partner might take on more caregiving responsibilities, and shared activities may decrease. Open, honest communication is essential. Talking about how you feel, your fears, and any changes in your relationship helps build understanding and emotional intimacy. Many couples find new ways to stay close, like cuddling, holding hands, or simply spending quality time together. Professional support can also make a big difference. Therapists and counsellors with experience in Parkinson's can help couples navigate changes in intimacy and offer strategies tailored to their unique situation.

5.2 HOW CAN FAMILY MEMBERS AND FRIENDS SUPPORT MY HEALTH AND WELL-BEING?

Family members can often help with daily activities such as meal preparation, medication management, transportation, and personal care tasks, helping you to juggle all the different activities in your daily lives. By offering empathy, compassion, and a listening ear, family members can also provide invaluable emotional support that helps navigate the challenges of Parkinson's with resilience and dignity. Your partner or children can also act as advocates and navigators within the healthcare system, accompanying you to medical appointments, facilitating communication with healthcare providers, and ensuring that treatment plans align with your needs and preferences. Involving your loved one in your Parkinson's treatment and care plans can foster collaboration, mutual support, and a shared sense of responsibility for managing the condition effectively. Support from existing social networks included emotional reliance, a sense of connection and cooperation (Pappa et al., 2017).

Open and honest communication within the family provides the basis for a strong social network that can act as the foundation on which you can build and open up to other social connections. Sharing thoughts and emotions and showing encouragement and compassion leads the way to deeper connections and models to others the way you would like to relate. Prioritising your partners' emotional needs is likely to make them feel valued and appreciated and more likely to reciprocate. Expressing your gratitude and celebrate small wins in your Parkinson's journey will encourage a relationship that is based on joy and love rather than hardship and sacrifice. In other words, treating others the way you would like to be treated is a good first step to build or re-build connection. Feeling guilty, avoiding difficult conversations, ignoring yours and others feelings are unlikely to help you connect with your partner or significant others. The more joyful our relationships are, the easier, enriching, and interesting our lives can be. Being proactive in building relationships and connection – and being curious about others and compassionate about their thoughts and feelings – not only allows us to know more about the people we share our lives with but also teaches us a lot about ourselves and enhances the way we think about things; this is a very useful skill to cultivate when Parkinson's throws unexpected challenges and symptoms that you need to navigate and think through.

Engaging in shared activities and hobbies fosters connection and strengthens bonds within the family. There are perhaps activities you enjoyed doing together before Parkinson's, if those are no longer available to you, perhaps think of ways you could adapt these activities or replace them. For example, if you enjoyed long-distance travel but it has now become difficult for you, what about traveling closer to home to unusual areas or places you've never been before. If you enjoyed going to restaurants but now the logistics make this activity less effortless and enjoyable, why not buy a cookbook for a cuisine you both enjoyed and try out a different recipe every week. Perhaps taking turns in cooking or cook together while chatting and enjoy a favourite drink.

There are also Parkinson's-specific activities that you could incorporate, and they can help you better understand Parkinson's. For example, you could attend Parkinson's local events or training, visit doctors together, and discuss the pros and cons of devices you could use to make life easier.

Recognise the importance of self-care for both you and your loved one, and prioritise opportunities for respite and relaxation. Arrange for occasional breaks or respite care to give your loved one time to recharge and attend to their well-being, knowing you are supported and cared for in their absence. Respite care services, volunteer assistance, or enlisting the help of other family members can provide caregivers with much-needed breaks and opportunities for self-care. Taking time for rest, relaxation, and pursuing personal interests is essential for replenishing energy and sustaining caregiving efforts in the long term.

By actively involving your partner in your Parkinson's treatment and care plans, you can strengthen your relationship, enhance communication, and empower each other to face the challenges of Parkinson's disease with resilience, compassion, and mutual support.

5.3 DO I JOIN A GROUP OR NOT?

Maybe you have pulled back from social interactions, not out of anger or sadness, but because it feels easier. Friendships can be one of the most meaningful parts of life, but Parkinson's can make navigating them tricky. Fear of visible symptoms like tremor or freezing, and efforts to conceal them, often lead to social withdrawal and increased isolation. Over time, this can erode relationships with friends, families, and romantic partnerships (Perepezko et al., 2019).

Joining a group can boost your social network; some people find these social engagements valuable. Parkinson's charities are helping individuals to organise group meetings in local community settings. Chatting with and engaging in activities encourages sharing experiences and information (Tuijt et al., 2020). This support was found important across the differing stages of the disease (Hellqvist et al., 2018). Social engagement can provide an opportunity to share knowledge, for example, what other people with Parkinson's had found helpful or what services they had used. Sometimes people in a similar situation are more honest with one another. 'You get with these people and you sit down and everyone is frank, you know, that is the one thing I really like about it. You don't find people pullin' their punches or anything, you know, they tell you what the problems are and how they have dealt with them, or in some cases, how they have not dealt with them' (Pappa et al., 2017, p. 91). The social interaction in general is more important than the activities themselves, as someone with Parkinson's reported in an interview study: 'It might not be the activity in itself, but the social interaction surrounding it. As I told you, we are friends meeting to prepare good food together. However, the cooking itself is less important; it is just getting together. That is what is important!' (Hellqvist et al., 2018, p. 3723).

If you already have a strong network that you can rely on, attending Parkinson's-specific groups might not be as helpful. On the other hand, you might have an already strong network but would also like to be with others who go through similar challenges to you, so being involved with a local group might help and complement your existing network (Pappa et al., 2017).

Recent studies show that social involvement with various people and activities can improve physical and mental well-being (Koetsenruijter et al., 2015). Whether attending a dance class for people with Parkinson's, talking with friends, or sharing experiences in an online support group, these interactions provide opportunities to strengthen your ability to manage the condition.

To sustain meaningful relationships, try to keep expectations realistic and accept people as they are. Remember that relationships take time to develop and effort to maintain, they can also grow and change over time just like a living organism. Be ready to share openly, taking time to listen and ask clarifying questions. Ask for help, and try to be as specific as possible and then openly show your appreciation and gratitude. Do not try to please everyone; take care of yourself and stay tuned to your own priorities. Be dependable and follow through on your commitments. In conflicts, avoid criticism; attack the problem, not the person. Recognise the rights of others to give their opinions. Approach relationships as a learning experience. Be creative; you may have to adapt activities you enjoy together.

Peer groups helped people accept Parkinson's and become better satisfied with their daily lives (Charlton & Barrow, 2002). However, some people might be frightened when seeing others who are going through the latter stages of Parkinson's, as they regarded others' situations as their future consequences. Sometimes it helps when a healthcare professional also attends the groups, provides some information, and facilitates a question-and-answer session. In the UK, you can find local groups, support, and social activities on Parkinson's UK's website. Add your postcode to see what is available in your area.

Joining a Parkinson's support group can offer meaningful social connection and practical advice. Many people find comfort and encouragement in meeting others who truly understand their experiences. Effective groups foster open communication, empathy, and shared learning. They often include educational resources, expert talks, and activities for people with Parkinson's and their caregivers. Whether in-person or online, these groups help build community, reduce isolation, and empower individuals and families to manage life with Parkinson's together.

5.4 WHAT ARE THE POTENTIAL BENEFITS OF SOCIAL ACTIVITIES, WORK, OUTINGS, AND HOBBIES IN MAINTAINING STRONG RELATIONSHIPS AND SOCIAL CONNECTIONS?

I had a video call with a lady with Parkinson's a few years back. She was considering taking part in one of my studies. One thing led to another, and we had a long conversation about life with Parkinson's. She had an early-onset diagnosis, was working part-time as a teaching assistant for reception children, and had two very young children. She was telling me how she was considering whether to keep her job or not as it was becoming increasingly difficult to do and perhaps she could do something else, more fulfilling, move to a different career, this led her to an internet rabbit hole where she was looking at other careers, looking to see how she can make a living from her hobbies, considering whether to become a stay-at-home mum and focus on her kids. Her very extensive online searches led to no answers, but she found my research course on mindfulness, and thought maybe that would help her clarify her thoughts. Fast forward to the end of the course, she still didn't have the answers she was looking for, but she had some tools to stay with the uncertainty and focus on what was important for her day-to-day.

Some people decide to leave their work after they have been diagnosed with Parkinson's, especially if they are experiencing anxiety and/or depression, have had Parkinson's for longer, and experience more functional and cognitive difficulties, in other words, when it is more challenging to fulfil the work demands (Timpka et al., 2023). People who remain in the workforce described goal adjustment, for example, changing their focus from career advancement to maintaining their current position (Habermann, 1996). There was no evidence that levodopa led people to rejoin the workforce. Professional activity following Deep Brain Stimulation was more often worsened than improved (Perepezko et al., 2019), but people's leisure performance was improved after Deep Brain Stimulation (Liddle et al., 2018).

Interview studies also revealed that leaving the workforce impacted other social roles and overall quality of life due to perceived loss of societal contribution and social contacts from work (Perepezko et al., 2019). Further, the types of activities in which people living with Parkinson's engaged tended to be more solitary and sedentary, such as reading or watching TV (Perepezko et al., 2019). Qualitative papers provided reasons for this shift to more sedentary activities, including people with Parkinson's giving up more physically demanding hobbies because of the disease or favouring more solitary activities because of the unpredictability of symptoms and embarrassment about symptoms (Perepezko et al., 2019).

After a Parkinson's diagnosis, individuals often experience shame regarding their symptoms, leading to their withdrawal from social activities and reducing social interactions (Carroll et al., 2022). This process can result in depression and social anxiety, affecting quality of life (Bognar et al., 2017).

People with Parkinson's mentioned that planning was crucial for maintaining social activities and navigating symptom demands (Thordardottir et al., 2014). Social and leisure role performance was improved for people living with Parkinson's who participated in activities with other people living with Parkinson's (e.g. tango class) (Perepezko et al., 2019). These classes naturally provided an opportunity for socialisation and meeting people with similar challenges.

Dance interventions, like support groups, provide a safe and non-judgmental space to connect with others facing the same challenges (Hashimoto et al., 2015). These programmes help participants feel accepted, share experiences, and gain new perspectives about the disease (Carroll et al., 2022; Hashimoto et al., 2015; Heiberger et al., 2011). People can discuss their symptoms openly instead of hiding them. Additionally, the music in dance provides a non-verbal way of communication and self-expression, which is particularly helpful for those with speech or expression challenges (Bognar et al., 2017). In short, dance offers a supportive space for connection, acceptance, and non-verbal expression, and those who participate often regain a sense of their social self and confidence in communicating with others. These benefits, in turn, help to reduce social withdrawal and increase participation in other activities (Bognar et al., 2017; Kalyani et al., 2019; Rios Romenets et al., 2015). The sense of belonging that dance interventions confer on people with Parkinson's boosts their motivation to continue, reinforces a beneficial cycle of increased participation and enhanced well-being (Heiberger et al., 2011; Ventura et al., 2016).

We may think of ourselves as an 'I', and the notion of an isolated self takes up much space in Western society. We all need safe, trusting, reliable, nourishing relationships. We need people who not only listen but also read between the lines and perhaps even gently challenge us. Prioritising relationships with family and friends can also help manage stress and feeling overwhelmed, as the focus is directed outwards. Participating in leisure activities and hobbies can promote relaxation, reduce stress, and improve overall well-being. Enjoying leisure time together allows us to unwind, recharge, and take pleasure in each other's company.

Social interaction will also enhance your emotional intelligence and increase the emotional support you receive. Social activities and outings create opportunities for empathy and validation. Sharing experiences, concerns, and feelings with others in a supportive environment can foster a sense of belonging and strengthen emotional connections.

FURTHER READING

Here are some resources on Parkinson's and relationships.

Parkinson's Foundation. (n.d.). *Dealing with relationship changes.* Retrieved June 4, 2025, from https://www.parkinson.org/living-with-parkinsons/emotional-mental-health/relationship-changes

Parkinson's UK. (n.d.). *Finding local groups.* Retrieved June 4, 2025, from https://www.parkinsons.org.uk/information-and-support/local-groups

Parkinson's UK. (n.d.). *Relationships, sex and Parkinson's.* Retrieved June 4, 2025, from 10525_Relationships Sex and Parkinsons_44pp_V4.pdf

REFERENCES

Agid, Y., Schupbach, M., Gargiulo, M., Mallet, L., Houeto, J. L., Behar, C., Maltête, D., Mesnage, V., & Welter, M. L. (2006). Neurosurgery in Parkinson's disease: The doctor is happy, the patient less so? *Journal of Neural Transmission Supplementum, 70,* 409.

Boel, J. A., Odekerken, V. J., Geurtsen, G. J., Schmand, B. A., Cath, D. C., Figee, M., van den Munckhof, P., de Haan, R. J., Schuurman, P. R., de Bie, R. M., & NSTAPS Study Group. (2016). Psychiatric and social outcome after deep brain stimulation for advanced Parkinson's disease. *Movement Disorders, 31*(3), 409–413.

Bognar, S., DeFaria, A. M., O'Dwyer, C., Pankiw, E., Simic Bogler, J., Teixeira, S., Nyhof-Young, J., & Evans, C. (2017). More than just dancing:

Experiences of people with Parkinson's disease in a therapeutic dance program. *Disability and Rehabilitation*, *39*(11), 1073–1078. https://doi.org/10.1080/09638288.2016.1175037

Buhmann, C., Dogac, S., Vettorazzi, E., Hidding, U., Gerloff, C., & Jürgens, T. P. (2017). The impact of Parkinson disease on patients' sexuality and relationship. *Journal of Neural Transmission*, *124*, 983–996.

Carroll, S. J., Dale, M. J., & Bail, K. (2022). 'Out and proud . . . in all your shaking glory' the wellbeing impact of a dance program with public dance performance for people with Parkinson's disease: A qualitative study. *Disability and Rehabilitation*, *45*(20), 1–12. https://doi.org/10.1080/09638288.2022.2122598

Charlton, G. S., & Barrow, C. J. (2002). Coping and self-help group membership in Parkinson's disease: An exploratory qualitative study. *Health & Social Care in the Community*, *10*(6), 472–478.

Fleming, V., Tolson, D., & Schartau, E. (2004). Changing perceptions of womanhood: Living with Parkinson's disease. *International Journal of Nursing Studies*, *41*(5), 515–524.

Gunnery, S. D., Habermann, B., Saint-Hilaire, M., Thomas, C. A., & Tickle-Degnen, L. (2016). The relationship between the experience of hypomimia and social wellbeing in people with Parkinson's disease and their care partners. *Journal of Parkinson's Disease*, *6*(3), 625–630.

Habermann, B. (1996). Day-to-day demands of Parkinson's disease. *Western Journal of Nursing Research*, *18*(4), 397–413.

Hashimoto, H., Takabatake, S., Miyaguchi, H., Nakanishi, H., & Naitou, Y. (2015). Effects of dance on motor functions, cognitive functions, and mental symptoms of Parkinson's disease: A quasi-randomized pilot trial. *Complementary Therapies in Medicine*, *23*(2), 210–219. https://doi.org/10.1016/j.ctim.2015.01.010

Heiberger, L., Maurer, C., Amtage, F., Mendez-Balbuena, I., Schulte-Mönting, J., Hepp-Reymond, M.-C., & Kristeva, R. (2011). Impact of a weekly dance class on the functional mobility and on the quality of life of individuals with Parkinson's disease. *Frontiers in Aging Neuroscience*, *3*, 1–15. https://doi.org/10.3389/fnagi.2011.00014

Hellqvist, C., Dizdar, N., Hagell, P., Berterö, C., & Sund-Levander, M. (2018). Improving self-management for persons with Parkinson's disease through education focusing on management of daily life: Patients' and relatives' experience of the Swedish National Parkinson School. *Journal of Clinical Nursing*, *27*(19–20), 3719–3728.

Kalyani, H. H. N., Sullivan, K. A., Moyle, G., Brauer, S., Jeffrey, E. R., & Kerr, G. K. (2019). Impacts of dance on cognition, psychological symptoms and quality of life in Parkinson's disease. *NeuroRehabilitation (Reading, Mass.)*, *45*(2), 273–283. https://doi.org/10.3233/NRE-192788

Kang, M. Y., & Ellis-Hill, C. (2015). How do people live life successfully with Parkinson's disease? *Journal of Clinical Nursing*, *24*(15–16), 2314–2322.

Koetsenruijter, J., van Lieshout, J., Lionis, C., Portillo, M. C., Vassilev, I., Todorova, E., Foss, C., Gil, M. S., Knutsen, I. R., Angelaki, A., Mujika, A., Roukova, P., Kennedy, A., Rogers, A., & Wensing, M. (2015). Social support and health in diabetes patients: An observational study in six European countries in an era of austerity. *PLOS One*, *10*(8), e0135079. https://doi.org/10.1371/journal.pone.0135079

Liddle, J., Phillips, J., Gustafsson, L., & Silburn, P. (2018). Understanding the lived experiences of Parkinson's disease and deep brain stimulation (DBS) through occupational changes. *Australian Occupational Therapy Journal*, *65*(1), 45–53.

Mavandadi, S., Dobkin, R., Mamikonyan, E., Sayers, S., Ten Have, T., & Weintraub, D. (2014). Benefit finding and relationship quality in Parkinson's disease: A pilot dyadic analysis of husbands and wives. *Journal of Family Psychology*, *28*(5), 728.

Pappa, K., Doty, T., Taff, S. D., Kniepmann, K., & Foster, E. R. (2017). Self-management program participation and social support in Parkinson's disease: Mixed methods evaluation. *Physical & Occupational Therapy in Geriatrics*, *35*(2), 81–98.

Perepezko, K., Hinkle, J. T., Shepard, M. D., Fischer, N., Broen, M. P., Leentjens, A. F., Gallo, J. J., & Pontone, G. M. (2019). Social role functioning in Parkinson's disease: A mixed-methods systematic review. *International Journal of Geriatric Psychiatry*, *34*(8), 1128–1138.

Rios Romenets, S., Anang, J., Fereshtehnejad, S.-M., Pelletier, A., & Postuma, R. (2015). Tango for treatment of motor and non-motor manifestations in Parkinson's disease: A randomized control study. *Complementary Therapies in Medicine*, *23*(2), 175–184. https://doi.org/10.1016/j.ctim.2015.01.015

Schupbach, M., Gargiulo, M., Welter, M. L., Mallet, L., Béhar, C., Houeto, J. L., Maltête, D., Mesnage, V., & Agid, Y. (2006). Neurosurgery in Parkinson disease: A distressed mind in a repaired body? *Neurology*, *66*(12), 1811–1816.

Singer, E. (1974). The effect of treatment with levodopa on Parkinson's patients' social functioning and outlook on life. *Journal of Chronic Diseases*, *27*(11–12), 581–594.

Soleimani, M. A., Bastani, F., Negarandeh, R., & Greysen, R. (2016). Perceptions of people living with Parkinson's disease: A qualitative study in Iran. *British Journal of Community Nursing*, *21*(4), 188–195.

Thordardottir, B., Nilsson, M. H., Iwarsson, S., & Haak, M. (2014). 'You plan, but you never know'–participation among people with different levels of severity of Parkinson's disease. *Disability and Rehabilitation*, *36*(26), 2216–2224.

Timpka, J., Dahlström, Ö., Nilsson, M. H., Iwarsson, S., & Odin, P. (2023). Time to workforce exit after a Parkinson's disease diagnosis. *npj Parkinson's Disease*, *9*(1), 72.

Tuijt, R., Tan, A., Armstrong, M., Pigott, J., Read, J., Davies, N., Walters, K., & Schrag, A. (2020). Self-management components as experienced by people with Parkinson's disease and their carers: A systematic review and synthesis of the qualitative literature. *Parkinson's Disease*, *2020*(1), 8857385.

Ventura, M. I., Barnes, D. E., Ross, J. M., Lanni, K. E., Sigvardt, K. A., & Disbrow, E. A. (2016). A pilot study to evaluate multi-dimensional effects of dance for people with Parkinson's disease. *Contemporary Clinical Trials*, *51*, 50–55. https://doi.org/10.1016/j.cct.2016.10.001

Zafar, M., Bozzorg, A., & Hackney, M. E. (2017). Adapted Tango improves aspects of participation in older adults versus individuals with Parkinson's disease. *Disability and Rehabilitation*, *39*(22), 2294–2301.

FINAL THOUGHTS: HOW TO LIVE WELL WITH PARKINSON'S?

Managing Parkinson's is not an all-consuming activity. Parkinson's does not necessarily have to take up every waking moment of your life. Making some time to sharpen your self-management tools, many of which are described in this book, will save you time and energy that you could spend on things that are truly important to you. Living well means spending time on things that matter.

Parkinson's is often thought of as a movement disorder, but as we've explored in this book, it is so much more than that. The challenges extend beyond tremors and stiffness to include changes in speech, facial expressions, sleep, mood, digestion, and how emotions are experienced and communicated. Each symptom, visible or invisible, tells a part of the story, and understanding them is the first step in managing them effectively.

Research is beginning to move us closer to finding a cure for Parkinson's. Various disease-modifying therapies are investigated that can offer ease of the symptoms and intervene in the disease process itself. However, these treatments are still in experimental phases. While pharmacological and surgical therapies will not cure Parkinson's, they represent important tools in managing the disease and improving quality of life. Treatments are becoming more

DOI: 10.4324/9781003484332-7

individualised, with greater attention to precision, safety, and patient goals. As research progresses, the hope is that these advanced therapies, especially when combined with holistic approaches like physiotherapy, mental health support, and lifestyle changes, will help people live better, fuller lives with Parkinson's.

Coming to terms with Parkinson's is not a linear journey; it is deeply personal, sometimes difficult, and often unpredictable. But within the uncertainty, there is also space for growth, resilience, and joy. You are allowed to grieve what you've lost, but you are also allowed to hope for what's still possible. By staying connected to who you are, leaning on support, and taking small, intentional steps each day, you can create a life that holds not just challenge, but connection, contribution, and moments of light. Parkinson's may be part of your story, but it does not define the whole of you.

Openness is the willingness to experience thoughts and emotions as they are, without trying to avoid or control them. Being open doesn't mean liking difficult experiences, but acknowledging them without resistance. When we don't spend time and energy to 'fight' experiences, feelings and thoughts, we have more time and energy to devote to what truly matters in life. When you catch yourself getting hooked in an experience, thought or feeling, and you replay it again and again, in your mind's eye, acknowledge it, maybe label it and let them pass like leaves floating down a stream. Even if the mind wanders, gently returning to this visualisation builds awareness and emotional flexibility. Practising this technique regularly, especially during moments of overwhelm, can help you regain clarity and stay anchored in the present. In short, openness means allowing uncomfortable thoughts and feelings to exist, without letting them dictate your actions, so you can live more fully in line with your values.

Recognising your values and aligning your actions with what truly matters to you can be a powerful way to support your mental well-being. Values are the guiding principles that reflect the kind of person you want to be and the life you want to lead, while goals are the concrete steps you take to move in that direction. By identifying your values, whether it is being a loving partner, staying active, or continuing to learn, you can create meaningful goals that give your life direction and purpose, even in the face of challenges. Reflecting on your daily activities through the lens of your values can help you see which actions bring you closer to the life you want and which take you away from it. Tools like the SMART goal framework (Specific, Measurable, Achievable, Relevant, Time-framed) can make your goals more achievable. It is also essential to anticipate and plan for barriers, such as Parkinson's symptoms or practical difficulties, so you can adapt your actions without losing sight of your values. Staying motivated involves taking small, consistent steps, seeking support, and reminding yourself regularly of what matters most. With clarity about your values, you can navigate the ups and downs of Parkinson's with a greater sense of meaning and direction.

Self-efficacy, the belief in your ability to take action and handle specific situations, plays a powerful role in managing life with Parkinson's. It is not just about what you can do, but what you believe you can do, and this belief shapes your motivation, persistence, and well-being. Confidence comes from several sources: your past successes (mastery), seeing others succeed (vicarious experience), encouragement from others (verbal persuasion), and how you interpret your emotional or physical state. Building self-efficacy through small wins, support from peers and professionals, and setting achievable goals can help you feel more in control and engaged in managing Parkinson's. Believing in your ability to handle your medications, exercise, or navigate social situations can lead to better outcomes, while doubt can lead to withdrawal and reduced quality of life

Managing pain doesn't always mean eliminating it. Many people living with chronic pain aim to regain a sense of control rather than complete relief. Working on thoughts and beliefs around pain can be effective. Avoiding activities out of fear of pain often leads to physical and emotional deterioration. Conversely, pushing through everything without acknowledging pain signals can also lead to further harm. Distraction through pleasant activities like reading or exercise can help, but sometimes that isn't enough. In such cases, acceptance, rather than resistance, can reduce the emotional layer of suffering. Accepting pain as part of life with Parkinson's doesn't mean giving up; it means redirecting energy away from fighting pain and towards meaningful action. Research supports that acceptance reduces suffering and increases functionality. Mindfulness, or staying present without judgment, helps the brain process pain differently.

In terms of fatigue, if you identify what exacerbates the fatigue and take care of those things, like stress, sleep, exercise and nutrition. Further, look into your all-or-nothing behaviours and avoid the 'catching-up-on-all-the-things-when-you-can' trap. Research evidence also suggests cognitive behavioural therapy, graded exercise, and stress management.

Some evidence shows that starting small and building habits in small steps gradually and steadily has a greater chance of success, as you won't be overwhelmed and can stick to new routines. Make your goals small and meaningful, choose activities that make you feel productive and satisfied, plan around your 'off' time, pace yourself, and be flexible. As with most things, the trick here is to do what feels right for you. You know yourself better than anyone else, and you will see if it will be best to start slowly or with all the habits you'd like to introduce to your life. If you want to start small, the first habit I'd suggest starting with is your sleep, as this impacts pretty much all other habits you'd like to build.

Good sleep is important for everyone, especially people with Parkinson's. Simple sleep hygiene rules can help you make the most of your sleep. There is no need to worry too much about a lack of sleep; it happens, it is not the end of the world. Make sure you have at least one activity built into the day so you feel tired and sleep at the end of the day, avoid napping too late or drinking coffee or alcohol close to your bedtime, and ensure the room you sleep in is dark and cool. If you find it difficult to fall asleep, it might be best to get up, read a book, do something else for a little while, and then get back to it, rather than spend time in bed tossing and turning. You might already know what helps you get a good night's sleep, so try to prioritise what is helpful for you every day. If you haven't found things that help you get to sleep, start reflecting every morning on the quality of your sleep and what you did before that, and that will give you clues of what you could do to help you get to sleep.

A healthy, balanced diet, particularly the Mediterranean diet, may offer neuroprotective benefits. It includes fruits, vegetables, whole grains, lean proteins, and healthy fats, and has been linked to slower disease progression and improved gut health. Caffeine and tea (especially black and green) may also have protective effects due to their antioxidant properties. Similarly, omega-3 fatty acids, genistein (from soy), and vitamins C, D, and E show promise in animal studies, though more human research is needed. These nutrients support brain health by reducing inflammation, oxidative stress, and neuron damage, but they should not replace prescribed treatments. Overall, good nutrition plays a vital role in managing Parkinson's, and combining various nutrient-rich foods may be more effective than relying on single supplements. Consultation with healthcare providers is important before making dietary changes or adding supplements.

Exercise is one of the most effective ways to manage Parkinson's symptoms, helping with everything from balance and strength to mood and motivation. Research shows that walking, strength training, flexibility, balance work, and aerobic activities all improve motor control, walking speed, physical functioning, and even reduce the risk of falls. Aerobic exercise, especially at higher intensities, may offer even greater benefits, like treadmill walking in virtual reality, which has been shown to reduce falls. Cycling and home-based exercise programmes, especially when made fun with gamification and coaching, also help with long-term commitment. Dance stands out as a unique and powerful form of movement therapy. Dance combines rhythm, music, and aerobic activity to help with motor symptoms and balance, while also boosting mood, motivation, and identity. Music-based movement taps into brain pathways that help synchronise movement and has even been shown to improve neurotransmitter activity, like dopamine and serotonin. Plus, it is fun.

However, despite the known benefits, most people with Parkinson's aren't getting enough exercise.

Motivation can be a major barrier. To boost your motivation, you can embark in a form of movement that also involves your partner, perhaps tango dancing or walking after dinner, group activities can also help you stay consistent with your exercise plans, or written exercise plans can help you work out the logistics of incorporating physical activity in your life and planning to overcome barriers.

Taking medication for Parkinson's is essential but it can also be complicated, frustrating, and at times unpredictable. Some days the medication works well, while symptoms return sooner than expected on others. This 'wearing-off' effect – when meds lose their impact before the next dose – can be unsettling. What helps? Knowledge and communication. Understanding how your medication works, how and when to take it, and what side effects to look out for can empower you to take control. Talk to your doctor – ask questions, voice concerns, and work together to find the best plan for *you*. Being included in these decisions makes a huge difference. Setting up systems to remind you to take the medication can also help. Ultimately, managing medication is more than just following a schedule – it is about building a routine that fits your life, understanding your treatment, and working with your care team.

One of the most important things you can do after a Parkinson's diagnosis is talk about it, especially with the people closest to you. Research shows that early, honest conversations with family can ease the emotional burden for everyone involved and create a stronger support network. But opening up isn't always easy. Many people hesitate to share how much they struggle, often trying to protect loved ones, especially children, from worry. The desire to appear 'fine' or to avoid being a burden can lead to emotional distance, even when family support is needed. Trying to hide visible symptoms like tremors or freezing can also lead to avoiding social situations. Over time, this isolation can strain relationships with close family, friends, and romantic partners. After Parkinson's, relationships can shift. One partner might take on more caregiving responsibilities, and shared activities may decrease. Talking about how you're feeling, your fears, and any changes in your relationship helps build understanding and emotional intimacy. Many couples find new ways to stay close, like cuddling, holding hands, or simply spending quality time together. Professional support can also make a big difference. Therapists and counsellors with experience in Parkinson's can help couples navigate changes in intimacy and offer strategies tailored to their unique situation.

By actively involving your loved one in your Parkinson's treatment and care plans, you can strengthen your relationship, enhance communication, and empower each other to face the challenges of Parkinson's disease with resilience, compassion, and mutual support.

Joining a Parkinson's support group can offer meaningful social connection and practical advice. Many people find comfort and encouragement in meeting others who truly understand their experiences. These groups – often organised by charities or communities – provide a space to share honest conversations, tips, and emotional support. For some, the social interaction is just as valuable as the activity itself. Even if you already have a strong support network, connecting with others facing similar challenges can be enriching. Effective groups foster open communication, empathy, and shared learning. They often include educational resources, expert talks, and activities for people with Parkinson's and their caregivers. Whether in-person or online, these groups help build community, reduce isolation, and empower individuals and families to manage life with Parkinson's together.

Taking an active role in managing your condition is not easy, at least at first. Hopefully, the suggestions in this book inspired you. Even if you find this process difficult, the good news is that we get better at things the more we practice. Part of practising is monitoring our progress and tinkering with our plans. Over time, having a full and meaningful life while keeping on top of illness challenges will no longer seem hard.

INDEX

For Product Safety Concerns and Information please contact our EU
representative GPSR@taylorandfrancis.com
Taylor & Francis Verlag GmbH, Kaufingerstraße 24, 80331 München, Germany

www.ingramcontent.com/pod-product-compliance
Ingram Content Group UK Ltd.
Pitfield, Milton Keynes, MK11 3LW, UK
UKHW021900051125
464716UK00007B/70